D1046563

LOOMIS'S ESSENTIALS of TOXICOLOGY

FOURTH EDITION

LOOMIS'S ESSENTIALS of TOXICOLOGY

FOURTH EDITION

Ted A. Loomis, M.D., Ph.D.

University of Washington School of Medicine
Seattle, Washington

A. Wallace Hayes, Ph.D.

Corporate Product Integrity
The Gillette Company
Boston, Massachusetts

ACADEMIC PRESS

San Diego   New York   Boston   London   Sydney   Tokyo   Toronto

This book is printed on acid-free paper. ∞

Copyright © 1996 by Ted A. Loomis and A. Wallace Hayes
Copyright © 1978, 1974, 1968 by Ted A. Loomis

All Rights Reserved.
No part of this publication may be reproduced or transmitted in any form or by any
means, electronic or mechanical, including photocopy, recording, or any information
storage and retrieval system, without permission in writing from the publisher.

Academic Press, Inc.
A Division of Harcourt Brace & Company
525 B Street, Suite 1900, San Diego, California 92101-4495

United Kingdom Edition published by
Academic Press Limited
24-28 Oval Road, London NW1 7DX

Library of Congress Cataloging-in-Publication Data

Loomis, Ted A.
    Essentials of toxicology / by Ted A. Loomis, A. Wallace Hayes. --
4th ed.
            p.   cm.
    Includes index.
    ISBN 0-12-455625-6 (alk. paper)
    1. Toxicology.   I. Hayes, A. Wallace (Andrew Wallace), date.
II. Title.
RA1211.L6   1996
615.9--dc20
                                              95-41426
                                              CIP

PRINTED IN THE UNITED STATES OF AMERICA
96   97   98   99   00   01   MM   9   8   7   6   5   4   3   2   1

CONTENTS

PREFACE

Toxicology is the study of the harmful actions of chemicals on biologic tissue. Therefore it requires an understanding of chemical reactions and interactions and of biologic mechanisms. The vastness of these subjects as well as the rapid day-by-day increase in knowledge that is directly or indirectly pertinent to these subjects precludes the possibility that any one mind could absorb and retain more than a small fraction of this information. However, it is evident that certain principles of modern toxicology are applicable to large numbers of chemicals and an understanding of these principles is essential for the development of an insight into the subject. These principles become basic to the study of toxicology and are the "essentials of toxicology."

When the first edition of this text was in preparation there were very few periodicals and reference volumes that were directly relevant to toxicology, whereas there are currently many excellent sources of information specific to the subject. Furthermore, these sources of information have become readily accessible through not only texts and periodicals but also computer databases. Because of this availability of information the current edition of *Essentials of Toxicology* employs a modified reference format. This book intentionally continues to be a concise presentation of the subject of toxicology as a basic science and considers toxicity of individual agents only in regard to their use as examples. Except for a few pertinent references directly in the text, references at the end of each chapter have been deleted and a separate chapter has been included to familiarize those readers new to this subject with the major sources of information in modern toxicology.

This edition of the book would not have been completed without the fortuitous joint interests and discussions between Drs. Loomis and Hayes together with the encouragement of Dr. Jasna Markovac, of Academic Press, all of which led to the current product.

We would be grateful to readers for suggestions, corrections, and criticisms that would make the next edition an even more accurate and worthwhile text.

Ted A. Loomis   A. Wallace Hayes

CHAPTER **1**

Introduction, Scope, and Principles

Early in the days of the development of civilization, man in his quest for food must have attempted to eat a variety of materials of both botanical and animal origin. Through this experience, it is likely that he found that certain substances, principally of plant origin, if taken into the body produced varying degrees of illness or caused death. Other materials served as a desirable form of food. Therefore, it would seem reasonable to believe that man soon recognized that there were harmful as well as beneficial consequences associated with taking materials into his body. All materials could be placed in two classes, one of which was safe and the other harmful. The word "poison" would be the term used to describe those materials or chemicals that were distinctly harmful to the body, and "food" would be the term used for those materials that were beneficial and necessary for the body to function.

This concept involving the division of chemicals into two categories has persisted to the present day and, as such, serves a useful purpose in society. It readily places certain biologic substances, and in fact all distinctly harmful chemicals, into a category which is accorded due respect. However, in a strictly scientific sense, such a classification is not warranted. Today, we certainly recognize that it is not possible to describe a strict line of demarcation, on one side of which may be placed the beneficial chemicals, and on the other side of which may be placed the harmful chemicals. Rather, it is much more reasonable, as experience has shown, to recognize that there are degrees of harmfulness and degrees of safeness for any chemical. Even the most innocuous of substances, when taken into the body in sufficient amounts, may lead to undesirable, if not distinctly harmful, effects. In contrast to this, the most harmful of all chemical agents can be taken into the body in sufficiently small amounts so that there will be no untoward effect from such chemicals. It is apparent that the harmfulness or safeness of a chemical compound is related primarily to the amount of that compound that is present in the body.

The single factor that determines the amount of harm that a chemical compound produces is the quantity of the compound that comes in contact with a biologic system. This quantity of the compound is commonly called the "dose." (Dose may be expressed using a variety of terminologies and is further discussed in the next chapter.) If a sufficient dose is taken into the body or comes in contact with a biologic mechanism, a harmful effect will be the consequence in the sense that the ability of that biologic mechanism to carry on a function is destroyed or seriously impaired. As the dose is increased from minimal to maximal levels, there is no sudden appearance of undesirable effects from any chemical agent. Rather, the response, whether it be beneficial or harmful, is a graded response and is related to progressive changes in dose. One of the most fundamental observations which may be made with respect to any biologic effect of a chemical agent is the relationship between the dose (or concentration) and the response that is obtained.

Thus, toxicology has developed into the study of the quantitative effects of chemicals on biologic tissue. Its focus is on the harmful actions of chemicals on biologic tissue, but in the quest for information regarding the harmful actions of chemicals, the toxicologist also acquires information which is relevant to the degree of safeness of the compound.

The word "toxic" may be considered synonymous with harmful in regard to the effects of chemicals. Many chemicals are so nonselective in their action on tissues or cells that they may be said to exert an undesirable or harmful effect on all living matter. Furthermore, such chemicals may be effective in rather small concentrations. In contrast to this, a given chemical may be sufficiently selective in its ability to produce harm that it acts only on specific cells. A chemical may be harmful to essential systems in several species of organisms, but capable of exerting its harmful effect only in a few of these species because of protective devices present in the resistant species.

When a chemical is said to be toxic, the average person interprets this to mean that it would have a harmful or undesirable effect on humans.

This may not be true when the toxicologist uses the word "toxic" and "toxicity," because it is evident that what may be considered harmful to one biologic specimen may be relatively harmless to another specimen; in fact, a chemical that is toxic to some organisms may be desirable as far as man is concerned. For example, a chemical could be harmful or even lethal to the mosquito, but relatively harmless, and therefore indirectly beneficial and desirable, to mankind. For this reason, man can make use of chemicals to his advantage solely because they may be toxic or harmful to some biologic mechanism. Therefore, if the term toxic or toxicity is used, it is necessary to identify the biologic mechanism on which the harmful effect is produced. Toxicity is a relative property of a chemical and may be directly or indirectly desirable or undesirable as far as man is concerned, but toxicity always refers to a harmful effect on some biologic mechanism.

Toxicity is a relative term commonly used in comparing one chemical with another. It is common to say that one chemical is more toxic than another chemical. Such a comparison between chemicals is most uninformative unless the statement includes information regarding the biologic mechanism under consideration as well as the conditions under which it is harmful. Therefore, toxicology is approached as the study of the effects of chemicals on biologic systems, with emphasis on the mechanisms of harmful effects of chemicals and the conditions under which harmful effects occur.

HISTORY

Modern toxicology is a multidisciplinary science and as such had to await the development of many of the natural sciences before it could become a quantitative field. Although many descriptions regarding the actions of poisons and antidotes were published prior to the nineteenth century, little of this information was based upon scientific studies.

The father of modern toxicology was M. J. B. Orfila, a Spaniard born on the island of Minorca, who lived from 1787 to 1853. Early in his career he studied chemistry and mathematics, and subsequently he studied medicine in Paris. He is said to be the father of modern toxicology because his interests centered on harmful (as well as therapeutic) effects of chemicals, and because he introduced quantitative methodology into the study of the actions of chemicals on animals. He was the author of the first book devoted entirely to studies of the harmful effects of chemicals. (Orfila, M. J. B.: *Traité des Poisons Tirés des Règnes Minéral, Végétal et Animal, ou, Toxicologie Générale Considérée sous les Rapports de la Physiologie, de la Pathologie et de la Médecine Légale.* Crochard, Paris, 1814-1815.) He was the first to point out the valuable use of chemical analyses as proof that existing symptomatology was related to the presence of the chemical in the body. He criticized and demonstrated the inefficiency of many of the antidotes that were recommended for therapy in those days. Many of his concepts regarding the treatment of poisoning by chemicals remain valid today, for he recognized the value of such procedures as artificial respiration, and he understood some of the principles involved in elimination of poison from the body. Like many of his immediate followers, he was concerned primarily with naturally occurring substances whose harmfulness was the focus of considerable folklore.

Although Orfila is considered the father of modern toxicology, Philippus Aureolus Theophratus Bombastus von Hohenhein, more commonly known as Paracelsus, also was a significant figure in the history of toxicology. Paracelsus (born in 1492 near Einsiedeln, Switzerland; died in Salzburg on September 24, 1541) formulated many then-revolutionary views that remain part of present day toxicology. He believed in the value of experimentation, a break with earlier tradition. Paracelsus, however, is best remembered as establishing the dose response when he stated, "All substances are poison; there is none that is not a poison. The right dose differentiates a poison and a remedy."

Modern toxicology borrows freely from several of the basic sciences. A knowledge of, and an ability to study, the interaction between chemicals and biologic mechanisms is predicated on a background in all of the basic physical, chemical, and biologic subjects. Toxicology borrows freely from the principles of chemistry, and more particularly biochemistry. It is dependent upon a knowledge and understanding of physiology. Familiarity with statistics and public health is fundamental to the study of toxicology. Pathology is a major part of toxicology, for a harmful effect from a chemical on a cell, tissue, or organism must necessarily manifest itself in the form of gross, microscopic, or submicroscopic deviations from the normal. The field most closely related to toxicology is pharmacology, for the pharmacologist must understand not only the beneficial effects of chemicals, but also the harmful effects of those chemicals that may be put to therapeutic use.

SCOPE OF MODERN TOXICOLOGY

In the United States in the past half century the teaching of toxicology has developed from a few incidental lectures given in courses presented in the Health Sciences and Public Health fields to the complete programs currently given in specific areas of the science. Occasionally one finds general introductory courses that are designed and presented in senior undergraduate programs. However, toxicology does not currently enjoy the status of an independent department within a college or university. Hence, the student of toxicology continues to study the subject in a fragmented fashion from a variety of sources. In medical schools, the teaching of toxicology is usually allocated to the pharmacology division of the school, where the subject is taught primarily as a description of the harmful effects on man of therapeutic agents and a few highly toxic substances. The diagnosis and treatment of chemical intoxication is taught in the clinics, and the clinical chemical methodology is taught in the departments of laboratory medicine. These sources of training are usually designed for the medical student but also are available to the student of toxicology. Courses in public health and preventive medicine generally include the statistical methodology and problems associated with exposure to chemicals in a working or domestic environment. Veterinary schools have excellent facilities for the study of the harmful effects of chemicals on livestock and pets. These schools instruct in the absorption, distribution, excretion, and metabolism of foreign chemicals and in the treatment of chemical poisoning in animals. Departments of fisheries and oceanography study and instruct in the effects of chemicals on marine forms of biologic tissue.

Thus, modern toxicologists are a collection of scientists from multiple disciplines who have a common interest in the harmful biologic effects of chemicals. There are the engineers and geologists who study the distribution of chemicals in the air, soil, and water. There are the chemists whose interest and ability rest in the detection and quantification of chemicals in biologic tissue. There is the pharmacologist whose interest is in the harmful effects of chemicals that are used as drugs. There are the industrial health physicians and public health officers who specialize in the control of pollution and the effects of pollutants on populations. There is the pathologist whose studies are concerned with the gross and microscopic effects of foreign chemicals. There are the veterinarians who are concerned with the effects of chemicals and plants, as well as feed additives, on livestock and pets. There are the marine biologists who are concerned with the adverse effects of foreign chemicals on marine life. Immunologists, geneticists, oncologists, and mutagenicists not only evaluate new agents for activity in their special areas of expertise but also use compounds that produce effects on these systems as tools in their studies.

The multidisciplinary nature of toxicology is one of its greatest strengths, for it brings the capabilities and techniques of experts in those sciences into the field of toxicology. It also allows for the practical and logical division of the subject into sections on the basis of the disciplines involved. Figure 1.1 shows three such divisions: Environmental, Economic, and Medical. The Environmental division includes the roles that engineering, environmental, and chemical specialists play in the identification and quantifica-

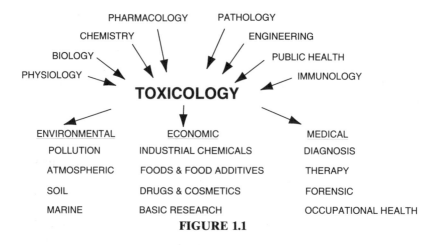

FIGURE 1.1

tion of natural as well as unnatural agents responsible for contamination (pollution) as well as transfer of chemicals between and within air, soil, and water. The Economic division involves the biologists, chemists, and basic medical scientists who identify and quantify the chemicals responsible for toxicologic problems in industry, in foods, and in drugs. It also includes the basic laboratory research programs that elucidate the chemical–biologic mechanisms responsible for harmful effects of chemicals on biologic tissue. The Medical division utilizes the capabilities of physicians and veterinarians for the diagnosis and therapy of chemical intoxication. As such it involves the forensic aspects of clinical toxicology, the pathology involved, and the public health consequences of chemically induced adverse health effects.

ENVIRONMENTAL TOXICOLOGY

The industrial revolution together with population growth has produced a complicated array of patterns by which chemicals are transferred from their sources into and within the environment. A simplified overview of these patterns is shown in Fig. 1.2. It shows that all chemicals eventually become waste and are translocated either as the original agent or as a transformed product of the original agent. Regardless of whether the original agent was man-made, was a product from biologic sources, or pre-existed in the soil, it can eventually reach the environment. The environment, composed of air, water, and soil, serves as both a supply source and a dump site for chemicals and their derivatives and translocates each agent

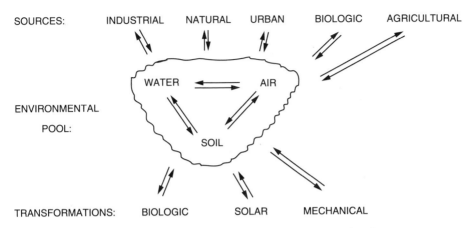

FIGURE 1.2 Waste chemicals and the environmental cycles.

within the environmental pool. Transformation products may be relatively more or less toxic as compared to the untransformed agent. The pool serves as an efficient system for diluting agents generally without showing partiality regarding the order of toxicity of various compounds. Hence dilution by the massive environment is a major mechanism by which chemicals supposedly disappear from existence and from importance in toxicology. Only when the pool is overwhelmed and the patterns of distribution fail, thereby leading to accumulation of agents at sites important to man's existence, does the system result in adverse chemical-induced effects on man. Some examples are the localized creation of smog over highly industrialized urban areas and the bioaccumulation of industrial waste products (e.g., methyl mercury) in fish consumed by humans.

Exposure to chemicals in the environment and the public health consequences are a continuing source of concern in toxicology. Because direct, reliable data regarding what ultimately happens to the large number of chemicals produced and used by humans are fragmented, there is concern about their persistence and possible accumulation in the environment. Some such agents do, in fact, accumulate, particularly in animals and aquatic forms of life which ingest them with food or water. Others undergo bacterial or biologic transformation to new chemical entities which also eventually reach the environment. Still others appear in the groundwater or soil where solar energy converts them to additional products. Others simply persist because of their high degree of stability. Although it is tempting to believe that the environment is sufficiently massive that it will ultimately dilute such agents to concentrations that have no biologic effect, this is clearly not true. Furthermore, the environment is not always a detoxication medium; for example, the chlorine which is added to drinking water will appear in wastewater, where it can react with organic material to produce chlorinated hydrocarbons, some of which are suspected carcinogens. This is only one of many reasons that nationwide monitoring of drinking water supplies has been conducted routinely since the early 1970s. Various water supplies have been shown to collectively contain minute quantities of more than 1000 chemical entities. The National Academy of Sciences (Safe Drinking Water Committee) has published 10 volumes on the subject of pollutants in drinking water, covering aspects ranging from the basic principles of water contamination to the potential health effects of contaminated water.

Although contamination of air and water presents major problems, contamination of soil by natural as well as man-made chemicals is considerably more complicated because of the complexity of the chemistry of soils compared to air and water. In addition, all soils contain microorganisms and their nutrients and by-products, as well as air and water; this allows for the transfer of contaminants between these environments. Every individual physical–chemical property of each agent is involved in facilitating or inhibiting the translocation of the agent within the environment. Ascertaining the final depot of waste chemicals and their products is central to understanding and controlling the potential for the occurrence of adverse effects on humans.

In spite of the large number of chemicals that appear as waste in the environment, the exposures that have occurred (with the exception of certain catastrophes listed in Table 1.1 and some examples of occupationally related tumorigenicity) have not been shown to be responsible for significant mortality in humans. There are reports of a positive statistical relationship between water quality and tumorigenicity in humans, but the risks appear to be at the minimum reliable levels of the procedures involved.

The sublethal effects associated with exposures of large populations to chemical wastes in the environment present a complicated diagnostic medical problem. This subject is considered further in Chapter 14. The uncertainties regarding potential hazards associated with environmental contamination necessitate continued scientific vigilance in order to safeguard the public health.

ECONOMIC TOXICOLOGY

Although toxicology is a very diverse discipline, its central concern lies in the evaluation of chemicals with the potential for harmful effects on

TABLE 1.1 Some Disasters Resulting in Chemically Induced Illness and/or Death in Humans

Date	Toxicity	Location	Compound	Source	Illness	Death
1930	Paralysis	U.S.	Tri-o-cresyl phosphate	Beverage contaminent	50,000	?
1937	Kidney failure	U.S.	Diethylene glycol	Solvent in sulfanilamide elixir	353	105
1951–74	Minimata disease	Japan	Methyl mercury	Containment in food (fish)	520	80
1956–60	Teratogenesis	Europe	Thalidomide	Sedative drug	8,000	?
1971–72	Coma	Iraq	Methyl mercury	Pesticide-treated grain	6,000	459
1976	Chloracne, liver damage	Italy	Dioxin	Factory explosion	700–22,000	?
1984	Lung damage	India	Methyl Isocyanate	Factory explosion	60,000	1700

Note. Data adapted from *General and Applied Toxicology* (Ballantyne, B., *et al.*, Eds.), Stockton Press, New York, 1993; and *Goldfrank's Toxicologic Emergencies* (Goldfrank, L. R., *et al.*, Eds.), Appleton & Lang, Connecticut, 1990.

man. Since it is a rare occasion that toxicity data are obtained initially on man, most information is derived from experimental animal studies, on the basis that animal data, properly qualified, are applicable to man.

Industry recognizes that it is essential for some toxicologic data to be obtained on every new chemical that is to be released to society; consequently, a company either has their own elaborate facilities and research programs or hires outside laboratories to estimate the toxicity of their products. Federal regulation agencies set requirements regarding the nature of toxicologic data necessary for chemicals that are added to foods. In a similar manner, data must be made available on all new (as well as existing) drugs to ensure that such therapeutic agents are not only effective but also safe.

Academia, as well as industry, expends considerable effort in determining the mechanisms of chemical–biological interactions. History has shown that an understanding of the mechanism of action of some highly toxic compounds can suggest concepts for the development of new drugs and newer, safer industrial chemicals. Although most toxicologic data are obtained via animal experimentation, considerable progress has been made in recent years in the development of *in vitro* toxicologic protocols.

The industries involved in production of chemicals, the agencies involved in the regulation and control of distribution of chemical products, and the laboratories involved in studying chemical–biological interactions all contribute to the acquisition of knowledge about the harmful effects of chemicals. These activities collectively compose the branch of toxicology that is identified in Fig. 1.1 as "economic toxicology."

MEDICAL TOXICOLOGY

Currently there are more than 100,000 chemical entities to which the general human population could be exposed. A student of toxicology could not be expected to be knowledgeable about the toxicity of even a small fraction of these. However, in spite of the multitude of chemicals that are potentially harmful, only a few have been adequately documented as causative of serious health problems in humans.

Periodically, catastrophic accidents expose large numbers of people to specific, known chemical agents. Examples of such accidents are given in Table 1.1. In these instances the consequences consist of not only deaths but also sublethal clinical effects. These incidents (and the publicity they receive) have made the general public justifiably concerned about insidious, sublethal, delayed, and harmful effects of chemicals to which they are exposed. In regard to sublethal illness from chemical agents, except for those catastrophic accidents, adequate documentation regarding causation is frequently lacking. Also, whereas some of the adverse drug or industrial chemical reactions have been well documented, others appear in the literature with inadequate documentation to support the role of the drug or chemical as the causative agent. Verification of possible chemical-induced illness presents a difficult problem to the clinical toxicologist (see Chapter 14).

In the disasters cited above, the chemical agents involved and the clinical consequences are clearly delineated. In the emergency rooms of modern hospitals as well as in the facilities of medical examiners the chemical involved in most lethal cases is determined by direct analysis. However, many deaths may be associated with the presence of specific chemical agents while the cause of death may not be reported in a form that allows it to be included in the statistical data on chemical-induced deaths. For example, an automobile driver intoxicated with alcohol may die in a collision, yet such a death would not be recorded as due to alcohol since the presence of the drug may be only coincidental. Similarly the death of a cigarette smoker may be due to lung cancer, but to record such a death as being due to cigarette smoke would be speculative. Conversely, a death that occurs in a residential fire may show that the death was due to carbon monoxide, but such a death would not be recorded as a chemical-induced death. Statistics that specify their data sources and limit their conclusions to the boundaries of the methodology used are the best sources of information on chemical-induced illness and death.

Regardless of the problems associated with the accuracy and completeness of data on chemical-induced morbidity and mortality, only through the acquisition of statistically evaluated data on these subjects can the magnitude of chemical-induced clinical problems be demonstrated.

Table 1.2 lists data showing that in 1970 and 1990 in the United States there were, respectively, 5299 and 5803 chemical-induced accidental deaths, or 2.6 and 2.3 per 100,000 population, and a similar number of chemical-induced suicidal deaths. Drugs and medicines were deemed to be responsible for about 3 out of 4 accidental deaths.

There are many more incidents in which chemicals cause sublethal poisoning rather than death. Table 1.3 indicates that in the United States in 1992 there were a total of 1.8 million inquiries regarding potential poisonings, from which 705 or 0.04% resulted in deaths. Approximately 50,000 or 2.7% of the total inquiries resulted in moderate or major consequences. Intentional exposure (that is, suicidal or abusive use) was involved in almost 11% of the exposures.

Table 1.4 summarizes a more detailed examination of the suspected causative agents responsible for the 705 deaths. It indicates that a variety

TABLE 1.2 Annual Deaths from Chemicals in the United States in 1970 and 1990

	Number of deaths		Rate/100,000 population	
	1970	1990	1970	1990
Deaths from accidents				
Drugs and medicines	2505	4506	1.2	1.8
Other solids/liquids	1174	549	0.6	0.2
Gases and vapors	1620	748	0.8	0.3
Total	5299	5803	2.6	2.3
Deaths from suicide poisoning (includes liquids and gases)	6584	5224	(3.2)	(2.1)

Note. From *Statistical Abstracts of the United States,* 113th edition, 1993, p. 98, except for numbers in parentheses which were calculated by the author (T.A.L.).

of chemical agents were responsible for the observed lethality. Drugs were responsible for 541 or 76.7% of the 705 deaths. Also, of all drug deaths, 391 or 72.3% were due to only 17 different drugs. Non-drugs were responsible for 164 or 23.3% of the 705 deaths, and about half of these deaths were due to only 10 chemical entities. Hence these data suggest that only a few chemicals or drugs (27) were responsible for a very high percentage of chemical-induced deaths.

Medical toxicology involves those disciplines that are concerned principally with the chemical identification, clinical effects, diagnosis, and treatment of chemical intoxication in human populations. In addition, medical toxicology involves the acquisition of information and the estimation of human risk associated with exposures of individuals as well as populations to chemical entities. This latter function includes the production of statistics on chemical-induced morbidity and mortality in humans.

FUNDAMENTAL PRINCIPLES IN TOXICOLOGY

From a fundamental and practical standpoint, the consequences of toxicologic effects on humans can be divided into two categories. One includes those consequences that are generally considered "irreversible," such as mutagenicity, carcinogenicity, teratogenicity, and of course death. The second category includes consequences that are "reversible," providing the initial damage is not overwhelming. Among these effects are organ damage,

TABLE 1.3   Poisonings Reported by Poison Control Centers in the United States in 1992

	Exposures		Deaths	
	Number	% of total	Number	% of total
Total	1,864,188	—	705	—
Consequence				
Unknown	873,718	46.9	—	—
None or minor	887,659	47.6	—	—
Moderate or major	49,693	2.7	—	—
Death	705	0.04	—	—
Site of exposure				
Residence	1,716,917	92.1	—	—
School	18,641	1.0	—	—
Workplace	46,602	2.5	—	—
Age group (years)				
<6	1,092,568	58.6	29	4.1
>50	7,270	3.9	201	28.5
Exposure				
Accidental[a]	1,624,424	87.1	107	15.2
Intentional[b]	199,950	10.7	541	76.7
Adverse reaction[c]	7,790	0.4	5	0.007

Note. Data are from 68 reporting centers serving a population of 196.6 million persons and are estimated to represent 78% of human exposures leading to poison center contacts in the United States in 1992. The data include telephone reports and treated patients and were condensed by the author (T.A.L.) from *Annual Report of Poison Control Centers Toxic Exposure Surveillance System* (Litovitz, T. L., Holm, K. C., *et al.*), *Am. J. Emer. Med.* **2,** No. 5, pp. 494–555, Sept. 1993.
[a] Misuse, occupational, environmental.
[b] Suicidal, abuse.
[c] Effects from drugs, foods.

such as damage to liver, kidney, or skin, and functional damage, such as respiratory depression, loss of consciousness, or convulsive effects.

Regardless of the category of any specific toxicologic effect, there are at least four basic principles that are generally applicable to all chemical-induced biologic effects of toxicologic interest.

1. The chemical must get to the effector site in a biologic system in order to produce a biologic effect. Although this may seem obvious, it is frequently overlooked in discussions of toxicity. For example, alcohol can produce harmful effects on humans, but a liter of whiskey in a bottle can have no effect (other than a psychologic effect) if it is not consumed; a liter of whiskey consumed in a short interval, however, contains enough alcohol to be lethal to the average adult. This concept can be extended to such scenarios as the asbestos in a building or the polychlorinated biphenyls in

**TABLE 1.4   Some Suspected Causative Agents Involved in 705 Deaths
Reported by Poison Control Centers in the United States in 1992**

Drugs			Nondrugs		
Category/agent	Number of deaths		Category/agent	Number of deaths	
Antidepressants	166		Fumes, gases, and vapors	36	
Amitriptyline		50	Carbon monoxide		24
Desipramine		22	Hydrogen sulfide		5
Doxepin		21	Chemicals (general)	19	
Imipramine		16	Cyanide		7
Nortriptyline		21	Strychnine		3
Analgesics	122		Insecticides	18	
Acetaminophen		63	Diazinon		5
Aspirin		35	Household cleaners	17	
Codeine		3	Hydrochloric acid		6
Morphine		7	Hydrocarbons	16	
Propoxyphene		7	Butane		9
Cardiovasculars	61		Alcohols	16	
Digoxin		16	Ethanol		10
Verapamil		28	Automotive Products	13	
Street drugs	61		Ethylene glycol		5
Cocaine		42	Methanol		5
Heroin		11	Miscellaneous[a]	29	
Methamphetamine		6			
Sedatives and hypnotics	49		Totals	164	79
Phenobarbital		9			
Antiasthmatics	36				
Theophylline		34			
Miscellaneous[a]	46				
Totals	541	391			

Note. Data in the Table were condensed by the author (T.A.L.) from the extensive data reported by Litovitz, Holm, *et al.* Annual Report of the American Association of Poison Control Centers Toxic Exposure Surveillance System, *Am. J. Emer. Med.* **11,** No. 5, pp. 494–555, 1993. The data include telephone reports and treated patients from 68 reporting centers.
[a] Miscellaneous includes categories with less than 10 deaths. For drugs this includes such categories as antihistamines, antimicrobials, anticoagulants, and topical preparations; for non-drugs, this includes adhesives, venoms, cosmetics, mushrooms, herbicides, heavy metals, etc.

the soil at a dump site. The physical–chemical properties, translocation, absorption, biotransformation, distribution, and elimination of chemicals are vital to an understanding of how an agent gets to a biological effector site.

2. Not all chemical-induced biologic effects are harmful. All therapeutic drug effects support this concept. This concept may be controversial in examples such as the increase in the amount (induction) of certain liver enzymes produced in experimental animals by many different chemicals and which may be either harmful or beneficial.

3. The occurrence and intensity of chemical-induced biologic effects are dose related; there is some dose below which no effect can be demonstrated, and there is a dose above which the agent is lethal. This principle is stated here because it is scientifically supportable. There is no conflict regarding the lethality of all compounds; however, the low dose, no effect clause is controversial since it is popular (but becoming less so) to describe those chemicals that induce irreversible effects such as cancer as creating a finite statistical risk, regardless of how small the dose may be.

4. Effects of chemicals on animals, if properly qualified, are applicable to humans. In order for this concept to be generally acceptable it should be recognized that there are quantitative differences in the effects of chemicals both between and within species. Also, the converse of this principle may be applicable in certain situations; that is, an effect may eventually be found to appear in humans which did not occur in animals. Usually such a finding is attributed either to differences between species in biotransformation systems or in biologic receptor sites, or to simple failure to examine for the effect in animal experiments. Consequently animal data must be "qualified" for it to be applicable to humans. Generally, whenever two species have similar biotransformation systems and physiological functions, those two species will respond similarly to chemicals.

CHAPTER 2

Numbers in Toxicology

It has been proposed that no chemical agent is entirely safe and likewise no chemical agent should be considered as being entirely harmful. This concept is based on the premise that any chemical can be permitted to come in contact with a biologic mechanism without producing an effect on that mechanism, provided the concentration of the chemical agent is below a minimal effective level. An implication of the concept is that all chemical agents produce a significant degree of undersirable effects if a sufficiently great concentration of the chemical is allowed to come in contact with the biologic mechanism. Thus, the single most important factor that determines the potential harmfulness or safeness of a compound is the relationship between the concentration of the chemical and the effect that is produced upon the biologic mechanism.

If one considers that the ultimate effect is manifested as an all-or-none response such as death of the biologic mechanism, and that a minimal concentration produces no effect, then there must be a range of concentrations of the chemical which would give a graded effect somewhere between the two extremes. The experimental determination of this range of doses is the basis of the dose–response relationship.

DOSE

The word "dose" as it is most commonly used refers to the quantity of a chemical involved or introduced into a biologic system in a unit period of time. Although the word dose has already been used several times in this text it should be recognized that it may appear in a variety of forms, the most common of which is weight of the chemical per unit weight of the experimental animal given on a single occasion (g/kg) or repeated daily (g/kg/day). A total daily dose may be divided into several doses administered at specific intervals (g/kg every 6 hr). As the need arises, dose may also be expressed as weight per unit body surface area, i.e., grams per square meter of body surface area per day.

In order for the word dose to be meaningful the route of administration or exposure also should be indicated. In animal experiments, the preferable route is by mouth (oral), in which case the chemical may be administered by stomach tube or may be dissolved or mixed with the animal's feed or water. However, several other routes are commonly used, such as intramuscular (IM), intraperitoneal (IP), topical, and intravenous (IV). When gases or vapors are involved the route of exposure is inhalation, in which case it is expressed as the concentration of the agent in the inspired air and the duration of exposure to that concentration. If an adverse effect is the objective of the experiment then the observation may be for a fixed time after the exposure. If death of the animal is the adverse effect that is measured, and exposure is for one continuous 8-hr interval with observation of the animals for 24 hr, then the dose is expressed as the 8-hr lethal concentration (LC-8 hr or LCt). In this latter example the quantity of chemical within the body of the animal is not known or implied in the term LCt; hence, it is an improper expression of "dose" but it is used for convenience. Also, when lethal aquatic experiments are conducted using fish, exposure is via the environment (water) and the procedure involves determination of the LCt, although exposure may be continuous for the duration of the experiment. Even in most *in vitro* studies in which cultured cells or tissues are exposed to chemicals, the lethal concentration (LC) in the nutrient solution represents the dose. In studies involving exposure to the chemical via a skin patch, the concentration of the chemical in the patch and the duration of exposure again determine the unit used to express the dose.

Some dosage forms carry specific meanings. One of the most frequent terms used in animal toxicology is the term NOEL for "no observable effect level." By definition this is the maximum dose used in an experimental protocol which produces no observable effect of any kind. It is always accompanied by the route of administration and the species involved (or type of experimental protocol). A NOEL may be misleading since it commonly represents only the highest dose from a series of widely spaced doses used in the experiment. If the sequence of doses had been more closely spaced, the experimenter may have found a different NOEL.

In clinical toxicology additional forms of dosage are common. One highly useful dosage form is that which identifies the amount or concentration of a substance in the atmosphere to which humans may be exposed without adverse health effects. Such a dose is called the threshold limit value (TLV) and is expressed as weight per cubic meter of air or as parts of chemical per million parts of air (PPM). TLVs are the clinical equivalent of the animal inhalation NOELs. The data for TLVs may be obtained from human experience or experiment and animal studies, and represent the opinion of an expert committee who are supplied with the animal and clinical data. Further modification of TLVs with the addition of "safety factors" by expert committees has led to the appearance of dosage terms used for regulatory and legal purposes. Such terms are PELs (permissable exposure levels), which represent the concentration of an agent in the atmosphere to which a person may be exposed without risk, and ADIs (allowable daily intakes), which represent, in the case of food additives, the amount that can be taken daily in the diet, even for a lifetime, without risk. These latter values may have little relation to any actual experimental data.

DOSE–RESPONSE RELATIONSHIPS

Under practical conditions, the biology experimenter finds that differences exist among the individual members of a supposedly homogeneous population of cells, tissues, or animals. The nature of these differences is seldom obvious and becomes evident only when the biologic mechanism is challenged, such as by exposure to a chemical agent. For example, a group of single cells such as bacteria or a group of whole animals such as inbred mice may be considered as uniform populations of biologic mechanisms, and as such may be exposed to a suitably selected concentration or dose of a specific chemical agent.

If the chemical agent is capable of producing an observable effect, such as death of the organism, or an effect from which the cells or animals completely recover in a period of time, then the dose or concentration of the chemical could be selected so that it would produce that effect. Furthermore, if the effect could be quantified, then the experiment would show that not all members of the group respond to the same dose or concentration of the chemical in a quantitatively identical manner. Rather, some of the animals would show an intense response, whereas others would show a minimal response to the same dose of the agent. Or, if the dose were properly selected, some of the animals or cells would die and others survive. Thus, what has been considered as an all-or-none response applies only to a single member of the test group and is found to be actually a graded response when viewed in regard to the entire group of members in the test. Such deviations in the response of apparently uniform populations of cells or animals to a given concentration of the chemical may be generally ascribed to biologic variation, a subject that is dealt with in detail in Chapter 6.

Frequency Response

Experience has shown that biologic variation in response to chemicals within members of a species is generally small as compared to biologic variation between species. Since one of the criteria of our experiment is that the response can be quantified regardless of the effect that is measured, then by further experiment each animal in a series of supposedly uniform members of a particular species may be given an adequate dose of the chemical to produce an identical response. The data obtained from such an experiment may be plotted in the form of a distribution or frequency–response curve. Such a representation for a hypothetical chemical agent is shown in Fig. 2.1.

The plot shown in Fig. 2.1 is frequently referred to as a quantal response curve because it represents the range of doses required to produce a quantitatively identical response in a large population of test subjects. The curve indicates that a large percentage of the animals that receive a given dose (Dose X) will respond in a quantitatively identical manner. As the dose varies in either direction from Dose X, some animals will show the same response to a lower dose, and others require a higher dose. Such a curve follows the laws represented by the normal Gaussian distribution pattern,

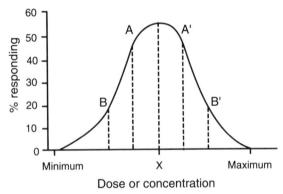

FIGURE 2.1   Hypothetical frequency–response plot following administration of a chemical agent to a uniform population of biologic specimens.

and is of considerable interest because it permits the use of statistical procedures applicable to such curves. The curve will be noted to have two main inflection points (A, A^1, B, B^1) on each side of the maximal frequency range. The dose identified as X is the *mean* dose, and the sum of all the animals responding to doses higher than the mean dose is equal to the sum of all the animals responding to doses of less than the mean dose. By definition, the area under the curve that is bounded by lines vertical to the abscissa from points A and A^1 encloses the total population corresponding to the mean dose plus or minus 1 standard deviation from the mean dose. Also, by definition, the area under the curve bounded by the vertical lines from B and B^1 to the abscissa includes the total population responding to the mean dose plus or minus 2 standard deviations of the mean dose. In actual practice, the true Gaussian curve is rarely, if ever, obtainable. Rather, a skewed variation of the curve is usually obtained as the best fitting curve for the experimental data.

Cumulative Response

In toxicology, frequency–response curves are not commonly used. Rather, it is conventional to plot the data in the form of a curve relating the dose of the chemical to the cumulative percentage of animals showing the response (such as death). Such curves are commonly known as dose–response curves. Figure 2.2 represents the dose–response relationship for two hypothetical compounds, the data of which may be obtained experimentally as follows: Groups of a homogeneous species, such as mice, are given

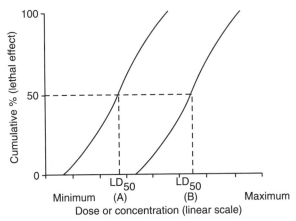

FIGURE 2.2 Hypothetical dose–response curves for two chemical agents (A and B) administered to a uniform population of biologic specimens.

the solution of the chemical by a specific route of administration. Only by experimentation can a dose be selected so that not all the animals die, nor do all of them survive. The initial dose may well be a dose so small that no effect is manifested by the animals. In subsequent groups of animals the dose would be increased by a constant multiple such as 2, or on a logarithmic basis, until ultimately a sufficiently high dose of the compound would be administered so that all of the animals in the group would die as a consequence of the exposure to the chemical. Thus, the only observation made in the experiment is that of death or survival of the animals. Under these conditions data would be obtained which may be plotted to give the results shown in graph form in Fig. 2.2. Figure 2.2 fulfills the implications of the concept presented in the initial paragraph of this chapter, that is, the dose of the compound may be sufficiently small so that no deaths occur. However, as the dose is increased, the typical S-shaped curve is obtained so that at sufficiently high doses, 100% of the animals die as a consequence of the exposure to the chemical.

Biologic experiments may be designed with the objective of determining the dose of a chemical required to produce any specific effect. When the experiments are done and a frequency distribution curve of the data is plotted, that curve is a visual representation of the differences among members of a test group of experimental subjects, a condition frequently referred to as "biological variation." Biological variation exists not only within species but also between species. When the data from the above experiment are plotted as a cumulative dose–response curve, the slope of the curve then becomes a visual and mathematical index of the differences among members of the test group. The measured effect need not be death of the animal but may be any type of biologic effect that can be quantified. The experiment need not be conducted on whole animals but may be conducted on a single cell system (such as a bacterial cell) or an isolated organ, tissue, or cell from any biologic system.

STATISTICAL CONCEPTS AND LD_{50}'s

Note that the major portion of the dose–response curve approaches linearity, and that insofar as this portion of the curve is concerned, the incidence of death is directly related to the concentration of the compound present. There is no question that the compound may be considered harmful or safe, depending upon the dose given.

The curve represents the concept by which the lethal dose for 50% of the animals is obtained. The lethal dose for 50% of the animals, which is commonly known as the LD_{50}, is that dose of the compound that will produce death in 50% of the animals. The LD_{50} is a statistically obtained virtual value. It is a calculated value which represents the best estimation of the dose required to produce death in 50% of the animals and is therefore always accompanied by some means of estimation of the error of the value, such as the probability range of the value. The limits of the probability range are arbitrarily selected by the experimenter to indicate that similar results would be obtained in 90 or 95 of 100 tests performed in a manner identical to that described. Several methods are available for the performance of such a calculation.

In the example given here, which is simplified for illustrative purposes, the LD_{50} is obtained from the curve by drawing a horizontal line from the 50% mortality point on the ordinate to where it intersects the curve. At the point of intersection, a vertical line is drawn and this line intersects the abscissa at the LD_{50} point. It is evident from the curve that information with respect to the lethal dose for 95% of the animals or for 5% of the animals also may be derived by a similar procedure. The LD_{84} (lethal dose for 84% of the animals) represents $+1$ S.D. (standard deviation) from the LD_{50}, and the LD_{16} (lethal dose for 16% of the animals) represents -1 S.D. from the LD_{50}. The percentage mortality may be converted to probits, which are numbers assigned to percentages so that 50% mortality equals a probit of 5, 50% mortality ± 1 S.D. equals a probit of 6 or 4, respectively, 50% mortality ± 2 S.D. equals a probit of 7 or 3 etc.

The statistical procedures that are commonly involved in toxicology are the same procedures that are used in the other biological sciences. The progressive improvements in the statistical methods and the development of computer technology as well as the lowering of the cost of the software and hardware has made it readily accessible to students and indispensable to scientists. The modern toxicologist needs mainly to understand which statistical procedures are applicable to his specific data and how to use modern computer technology to perform the mathematical chores involved.

POTENCY VERSUS TOXICITY

When data are obtained for two compounds, identified as compounds A and B, the curves representing the relationship between the dose and the incidence of death may be plotted as shown in Fig. 2.2. If the LD_{50} for compound B is greater than that of compound A, compound B may be said to be less potent than compound A. Furthermore, if dose and lethality are the only considerations, compound A can be said to be more toxic (harmful) than compound B. This would indicate that potency (in terms of quantity of chemical involved) and toxicity (in terms of harmfulness) are relative terms that can be used only with reference to another chemical. Therefore, one of the criteria that may be used to describe relative toxicities of two compounds is that of the relation of the doses required to produce an equal effect. However, as far as evaluation of the toxicity of a single compound is concerned, the absolute value of the LD_{50} may be in terms of a few micrograms or as much as several grams of a particular compound. If the LD_{50} is only a few micrograms for one compound, and is several grams for a second compound, the difference between the two compounds becomes highly significant. It is common practice to use the term "potent" for a chemical if the dose required to produce any effect is small, i.e., at most a few milligrams. Table 2.1 lists the LD_{50} values of a series of selected types of compounds and illustrates the range over which lethal effects can be induced in animals.

Because of the fact that some chemicals will produce death in microgram doses, such chemicals are commonly thought of as being extremely toxic (or poisonous). Other chemicals may be relatively harmless following doses in excess of several grams. Since a great range of concentrations or doses

TABLE 2.1   Approximate LD_{50} of a Selected Variety of Chemical Agents

Agent	Animal	Route	LD_{50} in mg/kg
Ethyl alcohol	Mouse	Oral	10,000
Sodium chloride	Mouse	IP	4,000
Ferrous sulfate	Rat	Oral	1,500
Morphine sulfate	Rat	Oral	900
Phenobarbital, sodium	Rat	Oral	150
DDT[a]	Rat	Oral	100
Picrotoxin	Rat	SC	5
Strychnine sulfate	Rat	IP	2
Nicotine	Rat	IV	1
d-Tubocurarine	Rat	IV	0.5
Hemicholinium-3	Rat	IV	0.2
Tetrodotoxin	Rat	IV	0.10
Dioxin (TCDBD)[b]	Guinea pig	IV	0.001
Botulinus toxin	Rat	IV	0.00001

Note. IP, intraperitoneal; IV, intravenous; SC, subcutaneous. LD_{50}'s are listed according to averages of nearest round figures from many sources. The principal sources are: Barnes, C. D., and Eltherington, L. G., *Drug Dosage in Laboratory Animals—A Handbook,* University of Calif. Press, Berkeley, 1964; *Handbook of Toxicology,* Vol. 1 (Spector, W. S., Ed.), W. B. Saunders Co., Philadelphia, 1956; Goldenthal, E. I. Compilation of LD_{50} values in newborn and adult animals, *Toxicol. Appl. Pharmacol.* **18:** 185, 1971.
[a] DDT, P,P¹ dichlorodiphenyl trichloroethane.
[b] TCDBD, 2,3,6,7-tetrachlorodibenzodioxin.

of various chemicals may be involved in the production of harm, categories of toxicity have been devised on the basis of amounts of the chemicals necessary to produce harm. An example of such a categorization, along with the respective lethal doses, is given below.

Extremely toxic   (1 mg/kg or less)
Highly toxic   (1 to 50 mg/kg)
Moderately toxic   (50 to 500 mg/kg)
Slightly toxic   (0.5 to 5 g/kg)
Practically nontoxic   (5 to 15 g/kg)
Relatively harmless   (more than 15 g/kg)

This classification serves a practical and useful purpose, but if the basis for ascribing the property of being "highly toxic" is because the lethal dose is small, then the question arises as to just where the line is to be placed to separate toxic from nontoxic chemicals.

Basically it is apparent that toxicity is relative and must be described as a relative dose–effect relationship between compounds. However, it is also apparent that the concept of toxicity as a relative phenomenon is true only if the slopes of the curves of the dose–response relationship for the compounds are essentially identical. It is possible that the slopes of the dose–response curves for any two compounds could be distinctly different, as are those that are shown for compounds C and D in Fig. 2.3. The LD_{50} of compound C is less than the LD_{50} of compound D. However, the reverse

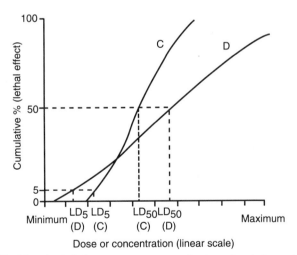

FIGURE 2.3 Hypothetical dose–response curves for two chemical agents (C and D) administered to a uniform population of biologic specimens.

is true for the LD_5's for the two compounds. If dose is the only consideration, it is apparent that compound C is less toxic than compound D because compound C has a higher LD_5 than compound D. On the other hand, compound C is more toxic than compound D when the comparison is made between the LD_{95}'s. It is therefore apparent that the slope of the dose–response curve may be most significant with respect to comparing relative toxicities of two compounds.

SAFETY VERSUS TOXICITY

Although the ultimate extreme in toxicity resulting from a chemical agent is manifested as a lethal effect, it is apparent that sublethal or reversible effects of chemicals may be harmful or undesirable, and therefore should be considered in any evaluation of chemicals with regard to their degree of harmfulness or safeness. Some of the commonly used drugs are the best examples of chemicals that can produce undesirable effects. Drugs that have as the basis of their action an ability to interfere with biologic processes are potentially harmful agents. This is particularly true if the primary action of the drug is concerned with a vital process. With such a drug, the therapeutic use of the agent is based upon obtaining a graded response from given doses which would result only in a desirable effect. If the desirable effect is exceeded, then the vital process would be sufficiently influenced so that a significant, harmful effect may result.

Many drugs have actions (side actions or side effects) in addition to the basic action of the drug. The side actions may or may not be undesirable, and as a rule a chemical becomes a drug only if the undesirable actions are not significant in comparison to the desirable actions of the drug. When morphine is given to produce analgesia, it also produces respiratory depression. When the anticholinergic agents are given for their effect on gastric motility, they also produce dryness of the mouth. Application of the antihistamine compounds or penicillin to the skin may initiate immunologic mechanisms resulting in sensitization phenomena which can be so severe that they result in death.

Undesirable effects of drugs are believed to be related to the dose of the drug. In the case of side effects of drugs, e.g., the morphine-induced respiratory depression or anticholinergic-induced dryness of the mouth, a relationship between intensity of the action and the dose of the drug is usually evident. That is, as the dose is increased, the intensity of the undesirable side effect also increases. In the case of sensitization to the drug applied to the skin, there may be little, if any, relationship between the dose necessary to produce a therapeutic effect and the dose necessary to induce sensitization, but there is usually a direct relationship between the dose, however small it may be, and the intensity of the sensitization response. The phenomenon of sensitization to a chemical involves an abnormal response to the chemical; this phenomenon is discussed in greater detail in Chapter 9. Therefore, toxicity or harmful effects from certain drugs necessitate separate consideration, for it is common practice to refer to one drug as being more or less "toxic" than another drug. However, toxicity from drugs is also a relative term, for it is also common practice to speak of one drug as being less toxic than another because the incidence or severity of side effects is less than for similarly useful drugs. The hope of the pharmacologist is to develop drugs which would be safe in all circumstances, but this is rarely, if ever, accomplished.

To a pharmacologist, the term "potency" means the relative dose of the drug that is required to produce an effect equal to that produced by a similarly acting drug. Thus, if two drugs are capable of producing a quantitatively identical effect, the drug that produces the effect with the lower dose is said to be the more potent of the two drugs. If the slopes of the dose–response curves for the two drugs are parallel, then the margin of safety between the two drugs may not be different.

The margin of safety to a pharmacologist is the dosage range between the dose producing a lethal effect and the dose producing the desired effect. This margin of safety is referred to as the therapeutic index and is obtained experimentally as follows: Two dose–response curves are obtained on a suitable biologic system such as mice or rats. One of the curves represents the data obtained for the therapeutic effect of the drug and the second curve represents the data obtained for the lethal effect of the drug. Figure 2.4 represents the data which may be obtained for a hypothetical drug in which curve A represents the cumulative therapeutic response and curve B the cumulative lethal response. The therapeutically effective dose for 50% of the animals (ED_{50}) is calculated from curve A, and the lethal dose for 50% of the animals (LD_{50}) is calculated from curve B. The margin of safety (therapeutic index) is represented by the ratio LD_{50}/ED_{50}. This is a useful concept in considering the margin of safety for practical use of the drug. Several authors have validly proposed that a more significant value would be derived from the ratio LD_1/ED_{99} as the most critical evaluation of safety of the compound. It is evident from Fig. 2.4 that if the lethality curve is shifted to the left so that it approaches the effective curve, the therapeutic index becomes a smaller ratio, the margin of safety is decreased, and the compound may be said to increase in toxicity.

When several drugs have similar actions and are used for similar therapeutic purposes, the drug with the greatest potency (in terms of therapeutic dose) is not necessarily either the safest or the most desirable drug. If no

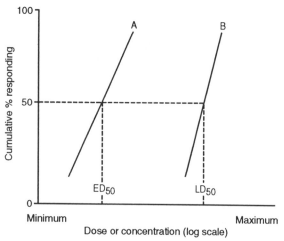

FIGURE 2.4 Hypothetical dose–response curves for a drug administered to a uniform population of animals. Curve A represents the therapeutic effect (for example, anesthesia) and curve B represents lethal effect.

other factors were involved, the drug with the highest therapeutic index would be the safest or least toxic drug, since therapeutic doses of it would be less likely to produce lethal effects. However, additional factors are always involved because, as already indicated, few, if any, drugs have but a single action. For example, since a margin of safety (or therapeutic index) is used to relate the therapeutic effect to the lethal effect, a similar margin of safety could also be calculated for the relationship between undesirable side actions and therapeutic actions. Such information is the aim of the drug toxicologist, who would like to develop drugs that have not only a high therapeutic index but also a high index in regard to freedom from all undesirable effects of the chemical.

The word safety basically implies the reciprocal of harmfulness. All chemical-induced biologic effects, some of which can be labeled as harmful, can be produced in the experimental laboratory. Harmful effects may be either reversible (sublethal) or irreversible (lethal). Each of these effects, including the absence of any effect, can be expressed in the form of a dose–response curve. Thus the overall picture of the safety as well as harmfulness of any chemical is dose related and can be graphically demonstrated as shown in Fig. 2.5. The figure shows that each effect would be represented by a curve with a specific slope and the range of doses applicable would be defined. If one first defines the nature of the harmful effect, then

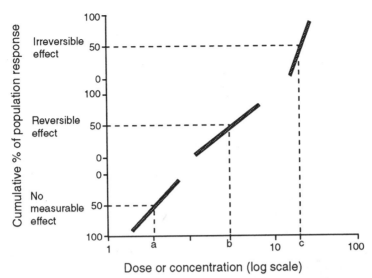

FIGURE 2.5 Hypothetical dose–response curves for "no measurable effect," "reversible effect," and "irreversible effect" from a single chemical substance. For illustrative purposes each curve is shown to have a different slope. The letters a, b, and c on the abscissa identify, respectively, that dose or concentration of the chemical at which 50% of the test population responds to each test parameter.

the order of safety or freedom from that effect in terms of dose becomes evident.

The numbers that are used in toxicology are derived from appropriately conducted experimental studies. These numbers are then subjected to statistical procedures that produce acceptable although virtual numbers. The virtual numbers are simply a concise form for expression of the results of an experiment and should be recognized as being applicable only to the specific initial experiment. However, in clinical toxicology it is acceptable to conclude that data from studies on animals, properly qualified, are applicable to humans. The final extrapolation of data from animal to man takes various forms, one of which is to simply add a safety factor of from 10- to 100-fold. Such a procedure results in numbers that are entirely virtual.

HYPERSENSITIVITY AND HYPOSENSITIVITY

In biology the application of statistical procedures to data that are experimentally obtained is a necessity, because only by such procedures can the range of the data be identified and validity of differences be established.

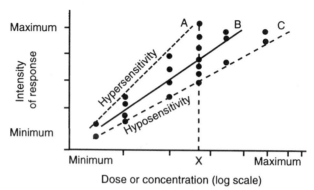

FIGURE 2.6 Hypothetical dose–response relationships for a drug administered to a uniform population of animals. Each point respresents response of a single animal.

However, the virtual nature of a statistically obtained value, such as the LD_{50} or ED_{50} of a chemical, tends to obscure an important concept in toxicology, the concept that there is no fixed dose or concentration of a chemical that can be relied upon to produce a given biologic effect in a population. This is evident from the frequency distribution curve shown in Fig. 2.1. It is common practice to speak of normals, hypersensitive members, and hyposensitive members of a population. The conditions that determine these categories of response are readily seen when the crude data for each contributing member are plotted on dose–response coordinates.

Figure 2.6 is a plot of a theoretical compound in which each point represents one item of contributing data. The figure shows that the mean dose–response relation exists (line B) for the normal subjects, and in order to include 100% of the contributions to the data, lines A and C represent the extremes of the data. Those subjects that deviate from the mean (line B) in the direction of line A are said to be hypersensitive to the chemical. Those subjects that deviate from line B toward line C are said to be hyposensitive to the chemical. The graph also indicates that following a given dose (or concentration), such as Dose X, the response may be below average or average in intensity, or the response may be maximum, *i.e.,* death of the biologic mechanism. The factors responsible for hypersensitivity of biologic systems to chemicals are an important part of the study of toxicology.

RESPONSE CONCEPTS FOR COMPOUNDS ESSENTIAL TO THE BIOLOGIC SYSTEM

Although the foregoing description of the direct relationship between the concentration of a chemical and any given response is correct for all compounds that are not normally present in the biologic system (such compounds are frequently called "xenobiotics," taken from the word "xeno," meaning foreign or strange), the concept does not hold for compounds that are normally present in the biologic system (that is, normal endogenous compounds). For example, the normal human will be in a state of health only as long as the body is supplied with nutrients and water as well as essential minerals and accessory food substances such as the vitamins. In the absence of these compounds as well as in the presence of an excess of the compounds, the human will develop undesirable effects. An example is shown in Fig. 2.7, which is a graph of the relationship between the concentration of total calcium in the serum and the response manifested in a human. According to the figure, there is a concentration range for calcium between 9 and 10.5 mg of calcium per 100 ml of serum which is necessary for normal function. This normal concentration of calcium as well as comparable normal concentrations of numerous other substances (i.e., glucose, hormones, sodium, potassium) is finely regulated by various homeostatic mechanisms. When there is a decrease in the level of the calcium, such as can occur when the body is not supplied adequate vitamin D or sources of calcium, the subject encounters muscle cramping due to the hypocalcemia. Conversely, when the calcium concentration is elevated above normal, the subject suffers from hypercalcemic malfunction of the kidney. Death can occur because of exceptionally low or high calcium concentrations in the serum of humans. In general, depletion of essential endogenous substances as well as excess of any essential endogenous substance results in toxicity to the subject. The specific nature of the endogenous substances that are essential to different biologic species will vary between species. This simple fact constitutes a mechanism that is extensively utilized as a means of producing death in an undesirable species by the use of chemicals. Some of the most widely used antibacterial drugs owe their action to an ability of the drug to prevent the bacteria from utilizing

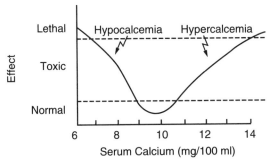

FIGURE 2.7   Relationship between serum calcium concentration and response in humans.

some essential nutrient; if that nutrient is essential only in certain species of bacteria, then only those species of bacteria will be affected by the antibacterial drug.

The conclusion that is reached is that xenobiotic compounds show simple, essentially linear concentration–response relationships, whereas essential endogenous compounds show biphasic concentration–response relationships.

Chemicals that possess selectively harmful mechanisms of action represent the greatest contribution of toxicology to science. Based on the theory that a chemical could be designed to be selectively toxic (lethal to a biologic mechanism that is present only in that species which it is desirable to eliminate) and provided the chemical is free of additional effects, such a compound would possess an infinitely high margin of safety for the biologic mechanisms which it is desirable to maintain. The development of chemicals as antibacterial agents, as pesticides, as herbicides, as anticarcinogenic agents, and as insecticides is rapidly approaching this ideal relationship between safeness and harmfulness of chemicals.

CHAPTER 3

Biologic Factors That Influence Toxicity

$\mathbf{I}$n order for a chemical to produce an effect on a biologic mechanism, a reaction (chemical or physical–chemical in nature) usually occurs between the chemical and some reactant chemical in the biologic system under study. It is also possible that an effect could be achieved solely on the basis of physical phenomena, such as a change in osmotic pressure, but such events are uncommon in toxicology. In all cases, the chemical agent under consideration must come in contact with some "reactant" chemical which is normally present at some location in the biologic system if a chemical reaction or interaction is going to occur. The reactant chemical is commonly referred to as the "receptor."

Even under nonbiologic conditions, a reaction between two chemicals takes place readily only if certain criteria are met by the reacting substances. First, the chemicals must be suitably selected and placed in physical contact with each other so that a reaction will take place. Second, the chemicals must be mutually soluble to some degree in some vehicle, because the addition of two substances in dry form usually does not permit sufficient contact between the reactants for a reasonable rate of reaction to occur. Third, unless a product of the reaction is removed, the reaction does not go to completion; rather, an equilibrium is obtained between the reactants and the products of the reaction. These criteria also must be met for a chemical reaction to take place in a biologic system.

Whenever a chemical is applied or administered to a complex system such as the human, unless the receptor is located at the site of application, the chemical must be translocated within the human to a receptor site if it is eventually going to produce an effect. For example, if a chemical is given by mouth it may be carried into the gastrointestinal tract, from there into the blood, and subsequently into the tissues and cells. Simultaneously while the processes of translocation are taking place, the chemical will be reaching incidental sites where it may be "chemically bound" (or "adsorbed") or "biotransformed" to new chemical entities. Furthermore, the initial chemical and its products will reach sites that serve to "eliminate" or "excrete" them from the body. Consequently chemicals that are taken into the body are eventually eliminated from the body. Different chemical entities will be present in the body for different periods of time, and since the mechanisms responsible for elimination collectively are usually dependent on the total body load, each chemical will show a specific half-life (time for the concentration of a compound in the body to fall by 50%).

The processes of absorption from some site of administration, translocation, and elimination occur simultaneously and regulate the presence and concentration of each chemical in the various compartments of the body. Although it is common to discuss absorption of an agent from the site of administration separately from translocation, the mechanisms responsible for absorption and translocation are similar since both basically involve passage of the agent across biologic membranes. The kinetics of these processes can be mathematically described and have developed into a branch of toxicology known as "toxicokinetics" (for non-drug chemicals) and "pharmacokinetics" (for drugs). These kinetics are discussed in detail in treatises devoted entirely to that subject. For the purpose of the current discussion, the kinetics involved in the translocation and elimination of a chemical agent supply the details of a fundamental concept in toxicology. This concept is that whenever a chemical is administered on multiple occasions over a period of time so that its rate of administration exceeds the rate of elimination, the agent will accumulate in the animal and thereby influence the degree of toxicity that is produced.

The biologic factors that influence the processes of translocation, elimination, and accumulation of chemicals in the body are considered in this chapter and the chemical factors are presented in the following chapter.

ABSORPTION AND TRANSLOCATION OF CHEMICALS

The complex biologic organism as exemplified by man is composed of a collection of organs, tissues, cells, and subcellular organelles, each of

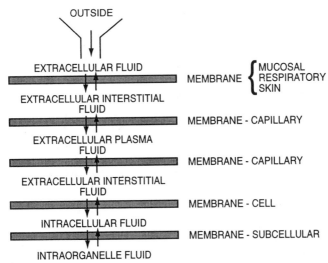

FIGURE 3.1 Schematic representation of membranous barriers involved in translocation of a foreign chemical from outside the mammalian organism to intracellular fluid in organelles.

which is protected from its environment by specialized coverings. These coverings give the structures their physical form and serve not only to protect their contents from temperature extremes, fluid loss, or mechanical insult but also to influence efficiently the free transfer of chemicals from access to their contents. In order for a chemical to gain access to a receptor that lies on or in an intracellular organelle, the chemical must effectively pass through a host of protective membranes.

Figure 3.1 is a schematic presentation of the membranous barriers that influence translocation of any chemical from the exterior of an animal to the intracellular compartments, that is, the organelles.[1] The process involves a series of translocation steps and increases the possibility of exposure of the administered chemical to large endogenous molecules, such as proteins, which may effectively bind and therefore functionally alter and remove the offending chemical from the animal.[2] Such a process also exposes the chemical to all parts of the body so that it is subject to excretion by the

---

[1] Organelles are subcellular compartments such as the mitochondrium, nucleus, and endoplasmic reticulum.

[2] In mammals, nonspecific binding of chemicals to proteins, such as albumin in the blood, effectively removes the chemical from the body by making it unavailable to react with a specific receptor. However, nonspecific binding is only temporary since it involves a readily reversible reaction; that is, as the concentration of the free drug diminishes with time there is a corresponding decrease in the concentration of the bound form. This reaction is shown in Fig. 3.2.

kidneys, by the respiratory tract, or even by the sweat glands. The molecule may be altered (biotransformed) by specific or nonspecific enzymatic systems present in the various organs. It may be deposited in storage tissues. Almost any reactive chemical that is administered to the organism is almost immediately subjected to mechanisms that may confine its translocation within the organism or terminate its existence as a free chemical (Fig. 3.2).

Since many foreign chemicals are capable of producing a specific effect on some biologic system or systems, such systems may be said to be the site or locus of action of the chemical. The locus may be strictly confined in one anatomic location within the animal, or it may be diffusely located throughout the animal. Since the effect of a chemical is a function of its concentration at the locus of action, it would be desirable to determine the concentration of the chemical at this site of action. In the intact animal, a limited amount of such information may be obtained by the use of agents tagged with isotopes which emit radiation energy or with heavy isotopes. More commonly the organ, tissue, or cells are prepared and analyzed by suitable chemical or physicochemical methods.

Once the existence and amount of the chemical at the effector site are verified, this information may be compared to the blood concentration of the agent at the same time. The blood is selected only because it is a readily available source of biologic sample material and the blood circulation represents the principal mechanism by which a chemical is carried to all parts

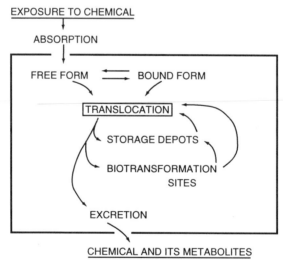

FIGURE 3.2   Schematic representation of the pathways through which a chemical agent may pass during its presence in the mammalian organism.

of the body. The ratio of the concentration of the agent in the tissue to the concentration of the agent in the blood at any given time would represent an index of the effectiveness or lack of effectiveness of the membranes to influence translocation of the compound. This technique may be used to demonstrate the translocation of a chemical between any of the systems of the animal. It is not uncommon that a chemical may pass readily from the gastrointestinal tract to the blood or from the lungs to all parts of the body except to the brain. Therefore, evidence indicating that a chemical agent readily passes through one membranous system in the organism does not necessarily mean that it will readily pass through all membranous systems in the organism.

Current concepts indicate that any chemical that does pass through membranes must do so by one or more of three possible mechanisms: (1) filtration through the spaces or pores in the membrane, (2) passive diffusion through the membrane through the spaces or pores or by dissolving in the lipoid material of the membrane, or (3) specialized transport systems which carry water-soluble substances across the membrane by a lipoid soluble "carrier" molecule, which effectively complexes with the chemical.

Fluid and its solutes are translocated between organs in the mammalian organism primarily by the blood and lymph circulation systems. The larger vessels of these systems serve only as conduits for transport of their contents to the various organs. It is only at the capillary division of the circulation system that fluid passes into and out of the blood. Capillary walls structurally consist of a single layer of flat epithelial cells held together by an "intercellular cement substance," through which it is currently believed that water and its solutes may be passively filtered. The process of filtration through a biologic membrane is not only a function of the hydrostatic pressure differential across the membrane, but also a function of the osmotic pressure differential on the two sides of the membrane. Shown in Fig. 3.3 are the forces that influence the transfer of water and water-soluble substances through the capillary membrane. At the arteriolar end of the capillaries, the hydrostatic pressure minus the plasma protein osmotic pressure within the capillary would have to be greater than the tissue hydrostatic pressure minus the interstitial protein osmotic pressure outside the capillary to permit the filtration of fluid from the lumen of the capillary to the extracellular interstitial fluid.

In contrast to this, at the venous end of the capillary the reverse condition would have to prevail, so that the quantity of fluid lost from the plasma at one end of the capillary is returned to the plasma at the other end of the capillary if the tissue is to maintain a constant fluid volume or weight. These conditions are met in the normal mammalian organism, and maintenance

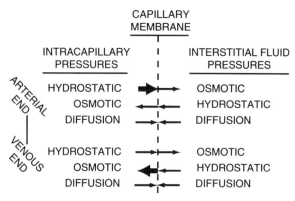

FIGURE 3.3   Schematic representation of the forces influencing transfer of water and water-soluble molecules through the capillary membrane in mammals.

of a constant body water volume is the result of the proper balance between filtration, hydrostatic pressure, diffusion, and colloid osmotic pressure on the two sides of the membranous barriers. If a filterable foreign chemical is present in the plasma and is only passively carried along with the filtered water, simple filtration would permit an equilibration to occur only between the plasma and the extracellular spaces in the tissue, but the filtration process could not account for the passage of foreign chemicals across the final cell membrane.

The mammalian cell membrane, which separates the contents of the cell from its environment, is composed of a thin layer of lipid or lipid-like material which is bounded on both sides by a protein layer, and the resultant membrane contains multiple pores. Most such membranes in mammals are of the order of approximately 100 Å in thickness, and the extremely small pores vary from 2 to 4 Å in diameter. Such a membrane is an effective barrier to the transfer of some chemicals into (and/or out of) the interior of the cell, and is an ineffective barrier to the transfer of other chemicals into (and/or out of) the interior of the cell.

Transfer of water-soluble foreign chemicals from extracellular tissue fluid to intracellular fluid must involve either the process of diffusion across the membrane in the direction of a concentration gradient or a transport mechanism which would permit transfer of the chemical through the lipoid portion of the membrane. Organic solutes of low molecular weight (such as urea, creatinine, and organic acids) pass freely across most cell membranes by simple diffusion, whereas ions such as sodium and potassium are selectively partitioned by the cellular membrane. In the latter case, the ions are selectively partitioned by an active transport mechanism involving energy expenditure to maintain electrochemical gradients on the opposing sides of the membrane.

The transfer of water across cell membranes probably occurs via the small-diameter water-filled pores in the membrane. Also, molecules that are sufficiently small may pass through the pores in the membrane. The pores of the membrane are relatively few in number per unit area of membrane. Therefore, lipid-insoluble substances that gain access to the interior of the cell have necessitated the development of a concept involving a special lipid-soluble carrier molecule, which is present in the membrane and is capable of combining with water-soluble molecules and carrying them across the lipid membrane to the interior surface of the cell, where the complex dissociates in the intracellular fluid. Thus, whereas some degree of water solubility appears to be desirable for the effective translocation of a chemical to the various organs in an organism, the cell membranes are only poorly permeable to such water-soluble substances. A water- and lipid-insoluble foreign chemical therefore would have difficulty gaining access to the intracellular fluid in an organism.

In normal humans, approximately two-thirds of all body water is intracellular. Therefore, if a compound is water-soluble and is carried freely across membranes, approximately two-thirds of the total amount of the foreign chemical in the body would be expected to be in the intracellular water. In contrast to this, the compound that could not pass the cellular membrane but was soluble in water would be partitioned in the extracellular water of the body. Thus, the addition of a foreign chemical, that is, a chemical not normally present in the cell, to an intact biologic system in its normal environment differs from the simple mixture of solutions of two or more chemicals. It is commonplace to observe that the amount of the chemical that produces inhibition of an enzyme system when tested on the isolated purified enzyme may bear no relation to the amount of the chemical necessary to produce a similar effect on that same enzyme when administered to the intact biologic cell; in fact, there may be a several hundred-fold difference between the two concentrations.

Some xenobiotic chemicals are so reactive with membranes that they are "captured" at the site of exposure to the chemical and little or no translocation takes place. The importance of this in toxicology is demonstrated by two highly reactive compounds, formaldehyde and methyl isocyanate, which are volatile at ordinary temperatures, thereby making inhalation the route of administration. Animal experiments have shown that these compounds can be efficiently removed from the air by the nasal mucous membranes during inspiration. Hence it is questionable whether even small amounts of these compounds are translocated to other parts of the body by inhalation.

RESERVE FUNCTIONAL CAPACITY

Organs basically have a reserve capacity to carry on their overall function. For example, approximately 50% of the liver of the dog can be chemically damaged or even surgically removed, and the remaining intact liver will carry on adequately to support at least the minimal requirements of the animal. Likewise, half the lung tissue in the rat may be removed without seriously endangering the life of the rat. Certainly, one kidney can be removed from any animal without harming the animal as long as a remaining kidney is in good functioning condition. Demonstration of chemical-induced damage to a living organ usually involves the use of one or more forms of tests designed to measure the function of the organ. Since it has been indicated that a large portion of the organ may be damaged before the reserve capacity of the organ is sufficiently diminished to render it functionally impaired, it is quite likely that function tests would not show small amounts of chemical-induced damage. In actual practice, this has been repeatedly demonstrated so that one must continue to rely on histologic or histochemical evidence to demonstrate the initial degrees of chemical-induced damage to an organ. Much research is currently directed at developing more specific and more sensitive tests of organ function in an attempt to detect small degrees of chemical-induced damage to organs. It is apparent that as long as the organ maintains a reserve (excess) capacity to carry on its overall function, such research attempts are ill directed unless a function of the organ is selected for which the organ maintains no reserve capacity, or unless the organ can be so stressed that it carries on the function at the maximal level.

The final concentration of the added chemical at various areas throughout the organ varies depending upon the ability of the membranes to be immaterial or to enhance or inhibit transfer of the chemical through the organ. In the process of the transfer of the chemical to a specific cell within the organ, the chemical must necessarily come in contact with nonspecific binding sites which functionally remove it from the system. Since it is postulated that a specific concentration of a chemical or its metabolites must be present if such a preparation is going to lead to toxicity of the organ, it is reasonable to conclude that some cells will be more or less affected than other cells for no reason other than the physical and biologic limitations placed on free transfer of the chemical uniformly throughout the organ. Such limitations may be practically insignificant if the chemical has the property of being freely transferable through the membranes. On the other hand, such limitations may be most significant and not easily overcome with a poorly translocated chemical, for it would mean that a constant concentration of a chemical would have to be maintained in contact with the organ for a sufficient time for some degree of uniform distribution of the agent to take place. Thus, an organ that has been insulted by minimal toxic concentrations of a foreign chemical agent on one occasion would not be expected to show the overall toxicity that would occur as a result of continuous insult by the same concentration of the chemical for an extended period of time.

ACCUMULATION AND STORAGE OF CHEMICALS IN THE ORGANISM

Exposure of a living biologic cell to a sufficient amount of a foreign chemical on a single occasion will lead to the presence of the chemical on and within the cell, provided the cell membranes allow its translocation within the cell. If the cell is then removed from the environment of the chemical, in time the organism will be free of the foreign chemical. The same mechanisms that are involved in the uptake of the chemical agent would be involved in the elimination of the agent from the cell, regardless of whether the cell is a single bacterial cell or one of a host of similar cells within an organ. In the case of the single bacterial cell, the act of removing the cell from the chemical-containing medium to a medium that is free of the chemical reverses the concentration gradient of the chemical, so that diffusion of the chemical could accomplish its elimination from the cell. In the case of the experimental animal, additional mechanisms of elimination are involved.

If the chemical passes into the circulatory system, it must then be eliminated from the circulatory system before the animal is free of it. If the chemical is in solution as a gas at body temperature, it will appear in the expired air from the animal; if it is a nonvolatile substance, it may involve excretion by the kidney via the urinary system, or it may be chemically altered by the animal and excreted via any of the mechanisms available to the animal, such as excretion in the urine, in the sweat, or in the saliva. The rate of elimination depends on the nature of the chemical and the mechanisms that are used to terminate the presence of the chemical in the organism. Generally chemicals that are metabolically converted by the animal to derivatives will have short lives within the body. An example is ethyl alcohol, which is metabolized at an approximate rate of 200 mg/kg/hr in man or the dog.

A chemical that is both metabolized and deposited in fat has a short life span in the blood and the nonfatty tissues; thiopental, for example, has a brief anesthetic action (15 min or less) following conventional single doses in man. This is because that portion of the drug which is in the blood rapidly undergoes conversion to nonanesthetic forms of the drug; the remainder of the drug is deposited in fat and muscle. Then as rapidly as the drug diffuses from the fat back to the blood, it is converted to inactive forms so that the blood remains essentially free of effective concentrations of the drug (see Fig. 3.4).

Many chemicals are selectively adsorbed on or combined with proteins or enzymes or even components of bone. Such chemicals may remain in the animal for years following a single dose. The drug Teridax (2,4,6 triiodo-3-hydroxyphenyl propionic acid) is so tightly bound to plasma protein that its half-life in the body is 2 1/2 years. Ninety-eight percent of the drug dicumarol is carried in the blood in combined form with albumin, where it is not available to produce an effect on cells or for metabolic attack by the animal. Atabrine is distributed in the dog so that the liver concentration of the drug after a single dose may be as high as 2000 times greater than the concentration in the plasma. The tetracycline drugs combine with components of newly formed bone in most laboratory animals so that reabsorp-

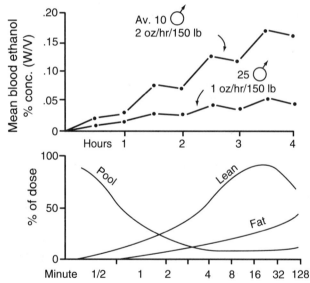

FIGURE 3.4 Upper graph represents, in the blood of human subjects, accumulation of ethanol following consumption of 1 or 2 oz of 100 proof whiskey per hour. First drink at Time 0 and one drink each hour thereafter. (Data from Forney and Hughes, *Clin. Pharmacol. Ther.* **4**: 619, 1963.) Lower graph represents translocation of a single dose of intravenously administered thiopental, a compound which is rapidly redistributed in the body and accumulated in fat. The figure shows initial translocation to the lean tissue and subsequent transfer to the fat. Data according to Price *et al.*, as predicted mathematically and compared with direct measurement in human blood and fat. (Price *et al.*, *Clin. Pharmacol. Ther.* **1**: 16, 1960.)

tion of bone must take place before the drug can be eliminated from the animal. The insecticide DDT (dichloro-diphenyl-trichloroethane) is stored in fat and remains in the animal for months. The organophosphate agents as exemplified by diisopropylfluorophosphate are effectively bound to and inhibit the enzyme cholinesterase, and hydrolysis of the phosphorylated enzyme is so slow that the enzyme remains inhibited for weeks.

Such sites of deposition, adsorption, or reaction of chemicals within the body limit the ability of the body to excrete them from the body. Such sites therefore act as effective storage depots for chemicals that otherwise may be so effectively metabolized or excreted that they would have only a transient existence in the body. Such sites of storage also effectively prevent the occurrence of high concentrations of the free chemical so that toxic concentrations of the chemical are not normally achieved until the storage site become saturated with the chemical. Thus, it would be reasonable to state that the potential toxicity of a chemical is influenced by the availability in the animal of an abundance of efficient nonspecific binding sites, or the presence or absence of efficient biotransformation mechanisms. Animals lacking such mechanisms would be very susceptible to rapid rises in concentration of the active chemical in the body, and since toxicity is directly related to the available active concentration of a chemical, such animals would be expected to be highly susceptible to the toxic action of these chemicals.

In general, single exposures of an experimental organism to a chemical result in uptake of the chemical by the organism and subsequent elimination of the chemical from the organism. The rate of elimination of the chemical is under the influence of the binding and storage mechanisms available for that chemical within the organism. Some gases may have half-lives within the body as short as a few minutes, whereas some strongly bound chemicals may exist in the body for years. Therefore, repeated exposures to a chemical in which the interval between exposure is less than the life of the chemical within the organism would lead to accumulation of that chemical in the organism.

Figure 3.4 consists of examples of accumulation of chemicals due to repeated dose (upper graph) and to translocation mechanisms (lower graph).

Chemicals that are bound to protein or to sites on the cell not involved in the pharmacologic or toxicologic response to the chemical represent large storehouses for such chemicals within the body. These bound forms of the chemical are generally not available for reaction with effector sites on the cells. However, it has been demonstrated that another chemical agent may displace the first chemical from the binding sites, making the first agent available in the free form. In this way the administration of a second drug could induce toxicity from the first drug; for example, the strongly bound sulfonamide drugs can induce hypoglycemic coma by replacing antidiabetic drugs which are bound to protein. Also, when patients who have received quinacrine (Atabrine) for the treatment of malaria are given primaquine, the primaquine displaces the quinacrine, which rapidly reaches toxic concentrations in the blood.

Compounds that accumulate in the body because of repeated frequent ingestion as contaminants of food have occasionally caused insidious harm to sizable populations of humans. Among the various chemicals involved in this type of clinical toxicology, methyl mercury is an outstanding agent that is responsible for at least eight separate episodes of tragedy directly affecting a total of over 8000 humans. Intoxication from this compound has resulted either from misuse, as food, of mercury-treated grain that was intended for seed purposes only, or because of industrial discharge of the compound (or related mercury compounds that are subsequently converted to the alkyl mercury by the action of bacteria) whereby it bioaccumulated in edible fish. The toxic manifestations of alkyl mercury (methyl or ethyl) intoxication in humans are loss of sensation, that is, paresthesia in the hands, feet, and the oral area, impairment of speech, and impairment of vision eventually leading to blindness. These effects are probably related to the effect of the alkyl mercury on brain cells. As far as the paresthesia is concerned, there appears to be a direct relation between the concentration of methyl mercury in the blood and the incidence and severity of the paresthesia. When a compound such as methyl mercury is taken by mouth as a contaminant of food, and when the particular food constitutes a staple item of the diet so that it is consumed daily, the compound has a good chance of accumulating in the body. Under these conditions of repeated intake by the oral route, methyl mercury is particularly prone to accumulate since it is very slowly eliminated from the body and it is very readily absorbed from the gastrointestinal tract. The half-life of methyl mercury is approximately 2 months.

Since it has already been demonstrated that toxicity is related to concentration of a chemical at effector sites and since accumulation of a chemical is a mechanism of increasing the concentration of a chemical in the body, compounds that tend to accumulate are prone to produce toxicity.

TOLERANCE

A poorly understood phenomenon in toxicology is that of "tolerance" to chemicals. Tolerance is the ability of an organism to show less response to a specific dose of a chemical than was shown on a prior occasion from the same dose. It is as if the organism becomes partially refractory to the effect of the chemical by virtue of previous exposures to the chemical. Tolerance could be due to any of at least three possible mechanisms. These are failure in translocation of the chemical to receptor sites, enhanced excretion or biotransformation systems, and elevation of the threshold of response at the receptor site. Currently there is little experimental evidence for or against the first mechanism. Biotransformation mechanisms are known to be altered by prior use of the same or related chemicals; this is discussed in the next chapter. The third possibility involves the creation of an altered receptor system through a change in the numbers or types of receptors involved.

In the toxicologic literature the term "tolerance" is frequently used incorrectly. For example, tolerance is different from resistance, as in the case of certain strains of rabbits which are known to be resistant to the effects of atropine because they have an enzyme in their gastrointestinal tract that inactivates atropine. Likewise, immunity that is developed to certain chemicals, such as the protein and polysaccharide toxins of bacteria, involves development within the animal of an antibody; this antibody then reacts directly with and inactivates the toxin on subsequent exposure so that the animal develops a resistance (immunity) and not a tolerance, to the toxin.

A significant component of the phenomenon of tolerance is that if a sufficient concentration of the chemical is presented to the organism, it responds by showing the conventional pharmacologic and toxicologic effects of the chemical. Tolerance is usually acquired over a period of time by exposure to an agent, but resistance to an agent may be acquired rapidly following only a few doses of the agent over a period of a few hours. In pharmacology this phenomenon is known as "tachyphylaxis." A good example of tachyphylaxis is the effect produced by the drug ephedrine. When ephedrine is administered to a cat or dog by the intravenous route it promptly produces a rise in blood pressure. With proper doses, this effect subsides within a half-hour, at which point a second dose will produce less effect. Each subsequent dose produces less and less effect until no response occurs, even if the dose is increased to virtually lethal levels. Hence, tachyphylaxis is not synonymous with tolerance to chemicals.

Tolerance occurs with most habit-forming drugs and in this respect acquires considerable significance in toxicology. In man as well as other animals repeated administration of morphine and related drugs results in tolerance to these drugs; a highly tolerant subject may require 20 to 40 times the usual dose of morphine in order to achieve the same degree of pharmacologic effect. However, even subjects with extensive tolerance to these drugs not infrequently take lethal overdoses of the drugs. Minor changes in absorption and translocation of morphine in the tolerant subject do not account for the tolerance. Rather, altered receptor sites in the brain, which have been described, appear to be responsible for the tolerance to morphine and related compounds.

Tolerance to many of the drugs that affect the human brain is accompanied by a compulsion to take the drug. If the compulsion is sufficiently strong so that the drug is taken repeatedly, a cycle of events leading to progressive increase in tolerance is established. Withdrawal of the drug may then lead to severe physical incapacitation and even death of such subjects. Such subjects are said to be addicted to the drug. Tolerance is a constant factor in addiction. The withdrawal effects that occur obviously constitute a type of harmful effect that is an exception to the basic concept that harmful effects of chemicals are directly related to concentration of the chemical present at the effector site. Withdrawal effects, as exemplified by delirium tremens in alcoholics or the hallucinating and convulsive effects in narcotic addicts, appear to be inversely related to the concentration of the drug in the tissue. In fact, administration of the drug relieves these effects. This represents perhaps the only condition whereby a type of harmful effect results from withdrawal of a xenobiotic chemical and is therefore inversely related to the concentration of the chemical at effector sites in the animal.

CHAPTER **4**

Chemical Factors That Influence Toxicity

$\mathbf{T}$he physical membranous barriers to translocation of a chemical in an organism are barriers only to compounds possessing specific chemical properties. Nonpolar compounds, as exemplified by ethyl alcohol, appear to pass readily across all biologic membranes in the living organism. The degree of ionization of a chemical in solution is a determinant of the ability of compounds to traverse membranes. Likewise, the solubility of the compounds in lipid material is an important factor with respect to transfer of chemicals across membranes. The chemical structure of a compound determines the ability of the compound to have a biologic action, and around this fact is built the science of structure–activity relationship (SAR).

Since all living tissues or cells are capable of carrying on metabolic processes, such cells possess the ability to alter (biotransform) many normally existing compounds as well as some foreign compounds with which the organism may come in contact. The biotransformation mechanisms are in many cases the result of enzymatic reactions which generate not only energy and products from nutrient chemicals, but also products of many foreign chemicals to which the tissue or organism may be exposed. Furthermore, certain laboratory animals as well as humans possess additional enzyme systems which may exist solely for the purpose of altering the structure of foreign chemicals. Therefore, the chemical factors that influence toxicity fall into two categories. The first category is composed of those chemical and physicochemical properties of compounds which individually and collectively determine the ability of the compounds to pass across biologic membranes. Such properties are important because they regulate the translocation of the chemical throughout the biologic tissue.

The second category comprises the chemical structure of compounds which enables them to produce specific actions on the tissues and to be susceptible to transformation by mechanisms present in the biologic specimen. Such biotransformation mechanisms are important because they may result in the formation of products possessing less toxicity than the parent compound or in the production within the organism of products possessing greater toxicity than the parent compound.

NONSPECIFIC CHEMICAL ACTION

Prior considerations of dose (or concentration)–response relationships indicate that all chemicals are potentially capable of producing harmful effects on living tissue. The mechanisms by which harmful effects are produced vary from a generalized destruction of protein to specific action on single-enzyme systems. Thus, strong acids or bases in high concentrations produce generalized destruction of all living cells, probably by precipitation of proteins with the consequent denaturation of the proteins and disruption of the integrity of the cell membranes. This nonspecific action is induced by concentrated solutions of all caustic or corrosive chemicals and involves partial to complete indiscriminate destruction of all parts of biologic cells.

A generalized overwhelming action of this type is no different from that which results from "cooking" or "burning" the tissue, so that such chemically induced effects are commonly referred to as "chemical burns." Such effects are produced not only by strong acids or bases applied in unphysiologic concentrations, but also by exposure to concentrated solutions of organic solvents, such as ether, chloroform, or carbon tetrachloride. The intensity of such nonspecific toxicity is directly related to the concentration of the chemical which comes in contact with the biologic cell. Generalized destruction of cells can be produced by any chemical that is sufficiently soluble in tissue fluids to gain access to the cells in high concentrations. In humans, these actions usually are limited to readily accessible tissues such as the skin, eyes, mouth, nasal membranes, and pulmonary airways.

SELECTIVE CHEMICAL ACTION

In contrast to the nonspecific, chemically induced destruction of cells from unreasonable exposure to chemicals, the majority of chemicals of interest in toxicology and pharmacology are sufficiently selective in their action that they produce harmful effects at specific sites in biologic specimens in concentrations far below those necessary to produce overwhelming destruction of cells.

Target and Receptor Concepts

Selectivity of action of chemicals signifies that within the biologic specimen substances (compounds) exist which are normal components of cells or cell membranes with which the assaulting chemicals are capable of reacting. Such normal components of cells may be referred to as "targets" or receptors for the assaulting chemical. The target may be very specific and vital to the function of the cell, and the chemical identity of the target is so altered by reacting with the assaulting chemical that it no longer carries on its function. The viability of the cell is thereby altered. For example, in the case of the mechanism of action of penicillin on susceptible bacteria the target for penicillin is a transpeptidase enzyme system in the bacteria that is involved in the synthesis of components of the cell wall necessary for its growth and stability. Penicillin reacts with and inactivates one or more of the transpeptidase enzymes, probably by an acylating reaction. The result is a weakening and eventual rupture of the cell wall of the bacteria, allowing extrusion of its contents into the surrounding medium with consequent death of the cell. Hence penicillin is most effective as a lethal agent to bacteria when they are in an actively growing phase. However, penicillin does not kill all forms of bacteria. This is probably because of structural differences between different strains of bacteria in their transpeptidase enzymes which alter their ability to act as targets for penicillin. Some bacteria can even destroy penicillin by producing penicillinase-type enzymes, thereby protecting themselves from the action of the drug. Thus penicillin is a selectively toxic chemical that affects only specific types of bacteria which have the transpeptidase system that is structurally specific to act as a target for the antibiotic drug.

In contrast to this, the target may be a protein or lipid which is not immediately vital to the function of the cell, and the reaction between the assaulting chemical and the target does not produce a direct alteration in cell function. In pharmacology, if the target with which the foreign chemical (or drug) reacts alters the function of the cell, such targets are given the general term of "specific receptors," signifying that a given drug intereacts or reacts with certain specific cell components. The same chemical may at the same time combine with, react with, or be adsorbed on extracellular proteins, but the function of the cells is not influenced by the product which is formed. Such combining sites on the proteins are referred to as "nonspecific receptors" for the drug.

In toxicology, a specific receptor is the cell component or components with which a foreign chemical interacts, thereby either directly or indirectly leading to the production of a harmful effect. When the receptor for a foreign chemical is known, it is not necessary to use such a noninformative term; rather, it is preferable to specifically identify the receptor. For example, the toxicologist may refer to the effect of mercury on the sulfhydryl groups of certain enzyme systems in which the sulfhydryl groups act as the specific receptors. The toxicologist recognizes that in the mammal one specific receptor for carbon monoxide is the hemoglobin molecule, that carbon monoxide has an affinity for hemoglobin, and that in reacting with hemoglobin it forms a hemoglobin–carbon monoxide complex which is not capable of carrying oxygen. Hemoglobin is therefore the receptor for carbon monoxide, and the kinetics of this reaction between carbon monoxide and hemoglobin have been well defined. However, in toxicology as in pharmacology, the exact receptor for many toxic chemicals remains to be defined.

The concept of specific receptors to chemicals is a useful concept in toxicology. Since the properties and structure of a chemical determine the affinity of that chemical for a biologic receptor, if the structure of one chemical entity is known and its receptor is known, then it is possible to predict the nature of the structure which is required to be more or less capable of reacting with the known receptor. Several useful drugs (for example, succinylcholine) and some of the most potent chemical agents known to man and of interest in toxicology were developed by prediction based on a knowledge of the chemical–receptor mechanism which was involved.

EFFECT OF IONIZATION AND LIPID SOLUBILITY ON TRANSLOCATION OF CHEMICALS

Many chemicals of interest in toxicology exist in solution in ionized and nonionized forms. Many drugs are weak organic acids or bases and only the nonionized forms are significantly soluble in fat. Since it has already been stated that the "pores" of the cell membrane occupy only a small part of the total area as compared to the lipid portion of the membrane, effective translocation of a chemical from extracellular fluid to the intracellular fluid should be facilitated by direct transfer of the agent through the lipid membrane. Current evidence strongly suggests that the nonionized, lipid-soluble form of an organic electrolyte is the predominant form capable of passing through the biologic cell membrane or the membranous barriers, which are composed of multiple cells.

The degree of ionization of an electrolyte in aqueous solution is dependent upon the pH of the solution. If the pH of an aqueous solution of an acid or base is adjusted so that the compound exists half in the ionized and half in the nonionized form, that pH is the acidic dissociation constant or pK_a of the compound. Conventionally, the dissociation constant for both acids and bases is expressed as the acidic dissociation constant or pK_a of the compound. An acid with a low pK_a is a strong acid, whereas a base with a low pK_a is a weak base. Conversely, a base with a high pK_a is a strong base and an acid with a high pK_a is a weak acid. At a pH above the pK_a of a compound, acids exist in aqueous solution mainly in the ionic form and bases in the nonionic form. Conversely, at a pH below the pK_a of a compound, acids exist in aqueous solution mainly in the nonionic form and bases in the ionic form. The pK_a of a compound may be derived from the Henderson–Hasselbalch equation as follows.

$$\text{for acids } pK_a = pH + \log \frac{\text{nonionized form}}{\text{ionized form}}$$

$$\text{for bases } pK_a = pH + \log \frac{\text{ionized form}}{\text{nonionized form}}$$

Therefore, if the pK_a of an acid or base is known and the pH of the aqueous solution of the compound is known, it is possible to calculate the ratio of the ionized to nonionized forms of the chemical in solution.

If two aqueous solutions of an electrolyte are separated by a biologic membrane that is permeable to only the uncharged molecules, in time a state of equilibrium occurs. At equilibrium the concentrations represented as the sum of the ionized and nonionized forms of the compound in each solution are identical if the pH values of the two solutions are identical, whereas the concentrations will be different if the pH values of the solutions are different. In the latter case, the concentrations of the electrolyte on the two sides of the membrane can be expressed as a ratio for any two pH values.

Since the pH on both sides of a cellular membrane in most organs of biologic specimens is essentially the same, if only the nonionized portion of the compound passes through the membrane, and if a compound is introduced to one side of the membrane, then it may be predicted that a compound that was highly ionized at that pH would fail to traverse the membrane as effectively as would a compound which was only poorly ionized at that pH. Compounds that exist at physiologic pH primarily in the nonionized state (provided the nonionized form is lipid soluble) would be expected to diffuse through membranes according to the direction of any existing concentration gradient until equilibrium is reached.

When a difference in pH exists on opposing sides of a membrane, a concentration gradient in regard to the nonionized moiety will be created so that when equilibrium is reached, the total quantity of electrolyte may be many times greater on one side of the membrane than on the other side. In the warm-blooded mammal, there are two sites at which the pH on the opposing sides of membranes may differ greatly. These are the mucosal surface of the gastrointestinal tract and the lumen of the tubules of the kidney. At these sites, the effect of pH on the ionization of organic electrolytes controls the transfer of the electrolytes across the membrane and therefore controls absorption of the electrolyte from the gastrointestinal tract and excretion of the compound by the kidney.

Shown in Fig. 4.1 is the proportion of nonionized to ionized forms of acetylsalicylic acid ($pK_a = 3.5$) in the stomach (at pH 1.0), in the intestine (pH 5.3), in the interstitial fluid or blood (pH 7.4), in acid urine (pH 6.8), and in alkaline urine (pH 7.8). At equilibrium, the concentration of the nonionized forms of acetylsalicylic acid in each fluid shown in the figure would be the same provided the membranes are permeable to the nonionized form of the drug. In order to reach equilibrium, the total quantity of drug present in each fluid will be different. Furthermore, that portion of the drug which is removed by nonspecific receptors such as protein would not contribute to the quantity of drug in each fluid as shown in the figure. The data in Fig. 4.1 are not corrected for protein binding. It is obvious that when a chemical is initially introduced into the stomach or the intestine, a concentration gradient for the chemical exists between the site of deposition and the other body fluids. If the chemical is capable of being absorbed,

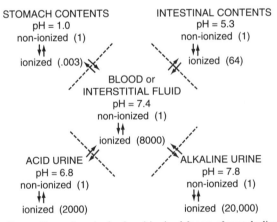

FIGURE 4.1   Proportions of nonionized and ionized forms of acetylsalicylic acid ($pK_a = 3.5$) in biologic fluids.

absorption progresses in the direction of the concentration gradient. If only the nonionized form is absorbed, the amount of the nonionized form determines the rate of absorption of the compound.

The direction of the concentration gradient for the ionized form of the drug across the mucosal membrane separating the stomach contents from the interstitial fluid would be highly favorable for rapid transfer of the drug from the stomach to the blood (Fig. 4.1). A similar, though less favorable, condition exists for the transfer of the drug from the intestine to the blood. Actual experimental results confirm the rapid absorption of aspirin from the stomach and intestine in humans.

When the kidney is forming acid urine, the concentration gradient of the nonionized form is in the direction of transfer of acetylsalicylic acid from the urine to the blood; under this condition the kidney would be expected to be a poor organ for excretion of the drug. However, if the kidney is forming alkaline urine, the concentration gradient for the nonionized form favors excretion of the drug from the blood into the urine. Actual experimental results confirm this concept (Fig. 4.2). The effect of alkalinization of urine on the excretion of acetylsalicylic acid from the dog, shown in Fig. 4.2, indicates that the excretion of acetylsalicylic acid is more than quadrupled by shifting the pH of the urine from 6.7 to 7.8. (Although

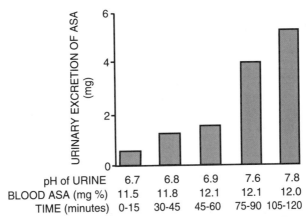

pH of URINE	6.7	6.8	6.9	7.6	7.8
BLOOD ASA (mg %)	11.5	11.8	12.1	12.1	12.0
TIME (minutes)	0-15	30-45	45-60	75-90	105-120

FIGURE 4.2   Effect of urinary pH on excretion of acetylsalicylic acid (ASA) by the kidney. Dog, male, 12 kg, hydrated with water (250 ml orally) 1 hr before the experiment. ASA (0.5 g orally) given 45 min before the experiment. ASA (50 mg) in 0.9% NaCl in water (150 ml) continuously infused during experiment. At 20 to 25 min $NaHCO_3$ (0.2 g) given intravenously. At 65 min $NaHCO_3$ (0.5 g) given intravenously. Urine collections made at 15-min intervals from an inlying urinary bladder catheter and each urine sample includes 50 ml water used to wash the bladder.

the above concept is valid for the purpose for which it is used, it involves an intentionally oversimplified version of the total number of mechanisms involved in urine formation by the kidney as well as the anatomic features of the kidney which permit formation of the blood filtrate and its ultimate appearance as urine.)

It is now well established that chemicals are readily absorbed from the gastrointestinal tract if the nonionized form is lipid soluble and if the pK_a of an acid is greater than 2 and for a base is less than 11. Chemicals are poorly absorbed from the intestine for several reasons if (1) the chemical is completely ionized in the intestine, (2) the nonionized form is not lipid soluble, (3) the chemical is destroyed by intestinal enzymes or microorganisms, or (4) the chemical is insoluble at the pH of the intestinal contents.

Provided they are organic electrolytes, chemicals that are strictly of toxicologic interest would be expected to follow these principles.

Chemical agents that do not undergo ionization or react with biologic fluids are absorbed and translocated according to the physical laws of diffusion and the solubility properties of the agent in water and lipids. In pharmacology, it is common practice to refer to the gaseous and vapor anesthetic agents (such as ether, chloroform, cyclopropane, nitrous oxide, ethylene, and divinyl ether) as substances that are nonreactive with tissue constituents simply because such agents generally are absorbed, translocated, and excreted from the body with little or no change in the chemical nature of at least 90% of the administered agent. In fact, except for minor losses of the compounds through the kidney and sweat, these agents are recovered primarily from the expired air of animals. Currently the mechanisms by which they produce anesthesia have defied precise description, but in general, anesthetic potency is directly related to lipid solubility.

Agents that are inspired through the pulmonary system diffuse across the pulmonary membrane according to Fick's law, which states that a gas will diffuse in the direction of a decreasing partial pressure gradient at a rate that is directly proportional to the diffusion coefficient and inversely proportional to the square root of the molecular weight or density of the compound. Thus the rate of diffusion of such agents into the blood of mammals is proportional to the partial pressure of the agent in the inspired air. This process of absorption of the drug from the air into the blood occurs at a sufficiently rapid rate so that equilibrium is reached by the time the blood makes one circuit through the lungs.

The concentration of the anesthetic agent is distributed to the tissues in direct proportion to their blood supply and their water and fat content (which determines the solubility coefficients for the various tissues). Nervous tissue has no special affinity for these anesthetic agents. Thus, as long as the anesthetic agent is administered to the animal, a shift in distribution of the agent in the various animal tissues will continue to occur until equilibrium is obtained throughout the animal. Under the actual conditions of use of anesthetic agents, it is doubtful whether the animal ever reaches total equilibrium only because the administration of constant concentrations of such agents is not continued for long periods of time. When administration is discontinued, the body eliminates the agent because the diffusion pressure gradients are reversed. The rate of elimination of these agents then is proportional to the partial pressures of the agents in the tissues, blood, and inspired air.

In toxicology, exposures to various gases and vapors may be continued for long periods of time, such as under the conditions encountered in the course of living in a contaminated atmospheric environment. The same principles that determine the absorption and translocation of the gaseous and vapor anesthetic agents would apply to any gas or vapor. In toxicology, it is possible that gaseous or vapor types of atmospheric contaminants would reach equilibrium in the body. When such agents are encountered in concentrations that do not give rise to acute signs or symptoms in the biologic specimen, there is some question whether chronic exposure to such chemical atmospheric contaminants can induce harmful effects. Such a question is usually answerable only by acquisition of data through experience. The American Society of Industrial Hygienists recognizes this problem and has published estimates of maximal allowable concentrations that may be considered safe for 8-hr daily exposure for approximately 500 chemical agents encountered in the atmosphere. A discussion of the basis for these estimates is given in Chapter 5.

Compounds that are inhaled and undergo ionization in biologic fluids would be expected to be absorbed, translocated, and excreted by the organism according to the conditions described for electrolytes.

BIOTRANSFORMATION MECHANISMS

Many foreign (xenobiotic) chemicals that are introduced into the body undergo chemical transformation, and this process is generally referred to as "metabolic transformation" or "biotransformation." The transformation processes are enzymatically induced and result in either the alteration of the parent molecule or the formation of products involving combinations of normally occurring substances and the parent molecule. Two categories of enzyme systems are known to exist in mammals. One category consists of enzymes that normally occur in the tissues and are responsible for transformation of normal endogenous chemicals in the tissues. The second category consists of enzymes that alter the structure of many foreign chemicals but have no established normal endogenous substrates.

A number of the enzyme systems that induce the tranformation of normal chemical substrates in the body are also active in catalyzing alterations of foreign chemicals that structurally are sufficiently similar to the normal substrate. For example, the nonspecific esterase-hydrolyzing enzyme cholinesterase not only hydrolyzes acetylcholine (a normally occurring neurohormone), but also will hydrolyze the local anesthetic agent procaine, as well as the muscle-paralyzing drug succinylcholine. Another example is the enzyme, monoamine oxidase, which is important in the metabolism of normally occurring biologic amines such as epinephrine and tyramine. This enzyme also oxidizes foreign short-chain amines such as benzylamine.

An enzyme system that is important in toxicology is that which has been extensively investigated in regard to the metabolism of drugs. These enzymes have become classed as "drug-metabolizing enzymes" and are frequently referred to as the "drug detoxication enzymes." These terms are misleading and should be discontinued not only because the enzymes catalyze transformation of many compounds that are not drugs, but also because the reactions do not always result in detoxication of the foreign compound. Rather, the toxicity of the product for many foreign compounds that are transformed by these enzymes is shown to be greater than that of the parent compound, by way of a process that may be termed "toxication" or "activation." These enzymes are referred to as drug-metabolizing enzymes only because of the common use of this term for identification of this group of enzymatic substances.

The drug-metabolizing enzymes consist of a group of enzymes that are present in many tissues but are particularly abundant in liver cells. Of the various components of the liver cells, the endoplasmic reticulum can be visualized with the electron microscope as filamentous-like structures of two types, smooth- and rough-surface filaments. It is the smooth-surface endoplasmic reticulum that contains the large proportion of the drug-metabolizing enzymes, whereas the rough-surface reticulum is concerned with enzymes involved in protein synthesis. When the liver cells are ruptured by homogenization of the cells, the endoplasmic reticulum undergoes fragmentation; these fragments can be separated by ultracentrifugation from the other parts of the liver cell. The fragments of the smooth reticular endothelium are then commonly called "microsomes."

Much of the information that has been obtained regrading the drug-metabolizing enzymes is based on *in vitro* studies utilizing the microsomal fraction of liver cells as the source of the enzymes. These microsomal enzymes are capable of catalyzing a variety of biotransformation reactions, among which are hydroxylation, dealkylation, deamination, alkyl side chain oxidation, hydrolysis, and reduction. The microsomal enzymes generally do not act on lipid-insoluble materials. In fact, they generally convert lipid-soluble compounds to less lipid-soluble compounds, thereby forming more polar substances that can be easily excreted by the kidney and by the biliary tract.

Shown in Fig. 4.3 are the types of metabolic transformation mechanisms important in toxicology. The figure is composed of mechanisms that have been shown to exist in several conventional laboratory animals. However, there are distinct variations in the pathways of metabolism for individual compounds, not only between species, but also within species. The figure includes an example of each type of metabolic transformation pathway. Several of the examples are of drugs and represent data obtained from studies on drug metabolism, which initially led to the demonstration of the existence of the enzyme system listed in the figure.

The microsomal material contains a membrane-bound, mixed-function oxidase system. It consists of a system enabling electron transport between compounds through the action of a variety of reductases plus a group of heme proteins that possess oxidase properties. The oxidase system is capable of attacking molecular oxygen (O_2) by reducing one atom of oxygen with the formation of water and incorporating the other atom of oxygen into a substitute xenobiotic chemical. The microsomal system more specifically operates as follows. It requires the presence of reduced nicotinamide–adenine–dinucleotide (NADPH) and molecular oxygen. NADPH reduces a component of the microsomes which reacts with molecular oxygen to form an active oxygen intermediate which oxidizes the drug. This may be viewed as a stepwise process involving initially the oxidation of NADPH by the action of a flavin enzyme (cytochrome *c* reductase); subsequently, in the presence of a reduced heme protein called P450, active oxygen is formed from molecular oxygen. P450 is so named because after complexing with carbon monoxide it shows maximal spectral absorption at 450 millimicrons. It is now recognized that there are several similar heme proteins (for example, P448) that have similar functions and which are identified by their maximal spectral absorption when complexed with carbon monoxide. The active oxygen oxidizes the drug. The reactions are listed as follows.

$$\text{NADPH} \xrightarrow[\text{reductase}]{\text{cytochrome } c} \text{NADP} + \text{H} \qquad (1)$$

$$(\text{Fe}^{3+})\text{P-450} + \text{H} \xrightarrow[\text{P-450 reductase}]{\text{cytochrome}} (\text{Fe}^{2+})\text{P-450} \qquad (2)$$

$$(\text{Fe}^{2+})\text{P-450} + O_2 \longrightarrow \text{``active oxygen''} \qquad (3)$$

$$\text{``active oxygen''} + \text{drug} \longrightarrow \text{oxidized drug} \qquad (4)$$

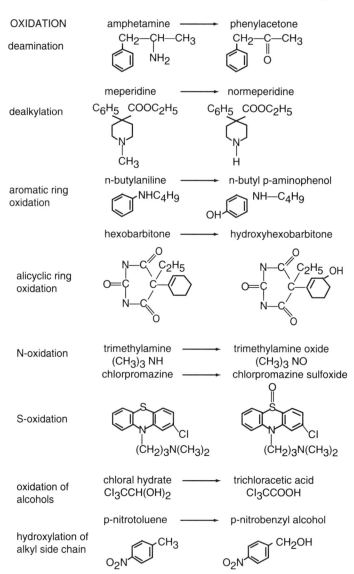

FIGURE 4.3   Some types and examples of biotransformation mechanisms in animals. The oxidation and reduction reactions are catalyzed by liver microsomal enzyme systems. The hydrolysis, acetylation, and conjugation reactions may involve enzyme systems from other tissues.

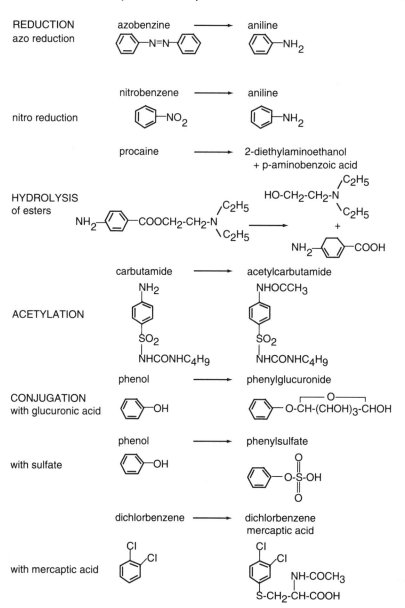

FIGURE 4.3 *(continued)*

The family of microsomal enzymes known as the cytochromes P450 also metabolize chemicals other than through oxidative and reductive mechanisms. In recent years much has been learned about the function of these enzymes and their action on xenobiotics through the discovery of selective inhibitors of members of this family of cytochromes P450.

Synthetic and Nonsynthetic Mechanisms

It is useful to divide the biotransformation mechanisms into two major types: (1) the nonsynthetic reactions involving oxidation, reduction, or hydrolysis and (2) the synthetic reactions involving generation of a product that is biosynthesized from the xenobiotic agent or its metabolite plus an endogenous agent or radical such as glucuronide or sulfate. One or both types of transformation may occur in the case of a single xenobiotic compound, and in various species the pathways for transformation may vary, depending on the availability in the species of the enzymatic system or endogenous products necessary for the reactions. Examples are seen in the fact that ethereal sulfate synthesis from phenols is a universal mechanism found in all species. The sulfation process involves activation of inorganic sulfate to an active sulfate which is 3 phosphoadenosine-5-phosphosulfate (PAPS) and serves as the sulfate donor. PAPS appears to sulfate aryl amines but not aliphatic amines. Glucuronide conjugation involves uridine diphosphoglucuronide, which probably represents a metabolically active form of glucuronic acid and has a normal role in conjugation of compounds such as the steroids, but which will also conjugate the salicylates, cinchophen, morphine, or codeine. Glycine conjugation occurs in most laboratory animals as well as in man, but glycine conjugation is replaced in hens by ornithine conjugation and in spiders by arginine conjugation.

An example of a foreign chemical that gives both the nonsynthetic and the synthetic types of reaction during metabolic transformation is one of the first compounds investigated, the diazo compound Prontosil. Prontosil, which was used initially as a dye material, showed antibacterial activity when administered to animals infected with hemolytic streptococci. It was soon discovered that the antibacterial activity was predominantly due to a metabolic product of Prontosil which was identified as sulfanilamide. It was then subsequently found that most animals were not only capable of reducing Prontosil to sulfanilamide, but also were capable of acetylating the sulfanilamide. Also, the acetylated compound was ineffective as an antibacterial agent. This series of transformation steps follows.

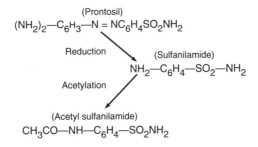

The metabolism of Prontosil serves as an example of several basic concepts of toxicology:

1. In regard to antibacterial activity, the first transformation reaction leads to activation of the compound, but the second reaction leads to inactivation of the compound. In the intact animal the first reaction takes place at a rate which exceeds that of the second reaction, thereby leading to accumulation of concentrations of sulfanilamide so that antibacterial activity is present in the animal. Had this not been the case, the mechanism of antibacterial action of Prontosil in all probability would have been over-looked. Many sequential transformation mechanisms lead to the formation of intermediate products, which exist as transient or only hypothetical products and would have to be extremely potent to have any significant toxicologic effect on the organism.

2. In regard to toxicologic effect on the host and in regard to acute lethal toxicity, the first step in the metabolism of Prontosil may be said to lead to the formation of a more toxic compound than the parent compound; the second step in the metabolism of Prontosil may be said to lead to the formation of a less toxic compound. However, in actual practice, Prontosil (or its metabolic products, sulfanilamide, and acetylsulfanilamide) produce several toxicologic effects which are not necessarily lethal. For example, in man sulfanilamide induces the formation of methemoglobin; it inhibits carbonic anhydrase, and it may produce fever, skin rashes, or blood cell dyscrasias. Since sulfanilamide is a metabolic product of Prontosil, some of these toxicities are induced by administration of the parent compound. In animals (the dog is an exception since it does not acetylate sulfanilamide) acetyl sulfanilamide is prone to precipitate in the kidney tubules, owing to its relative insolubility in urine as compared to sulfanilamide or Prontosil, and can obstruct the flow of urine. Therefore, as far as the host animal is concerned, both the first and second steps in metabolic transformation of Prontosil lead to the formation of products with some form of toxicity greater than that of the original compound.

In another example, understanding the pathways of metabolism of the analgesic drug acetaminophen helps to explain the mechanisms responsible for the hepatic toxicity of overdoses of that drug. Figure 4.4 shows these pathways. Following ordinary doses of acetaminophen in humans a portion of the drug undergoes conjugation with glucuronide and sulfate and the conjugates are then excreted in the urine. Simultaneously, a major portion of the drug is biotransformed via cytochrome P450 oxidative metabolism to form reactive metabolites which combine with hepatic glutathione and are converted to mercapturic acid derivatives. These are also excreted in the urine. Large doses of acetaminophen deplete the liver of its stores of glutathione, thereby allowing the reactive metabolites of acetaminophen to covalently bind to various liver cell proteins. This leads to death of the liver cells. Although the above sequence of reactions does not identify the ultimate "toxicant," clearly the depletion of glutathione stores is the critical problem leading to the hepatic cell death. Also it is now recognized that replacement of the thiol glutathione with a similar thiol, *n*-acetylcysteine, effectively reduces acetaminophen hepatic toxicity. (See Chapt. 11 on antidotal therapy.)

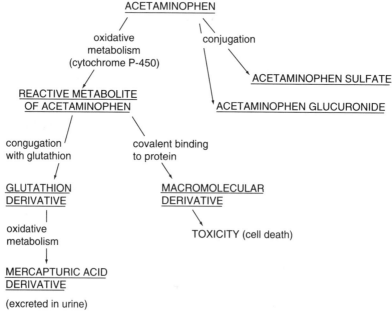

FIGURE 4.4   Acetaminophen metabolism and probable mechanism of hepatic toxicity.

It is now evident that determination of the toxicity of any compound which is metabolically transformed is in essence the determination of the toxicity of the parent compound and its metabolites. In fact, some of the most widely used pesticides are not effective pesticides and have low orders of toxicity to a host animal until they are metabolically transformed in the host to an active substance. A good example is the conversion of Parathion to Paraoxon. It is possible that parent compounds may exist for such a short period of time in the biologic organism that their usefulness as therapeutic agents is extremely limited. Such mechanisms help us to understand the difficulties encountered in transposing data that are acquired from *in vitro* observations of effects of chemicals to the intact animal.

There are many instances in which metabolic conversion of a chemical results in the formation of products that are more toxic than the original compound (Table 4.1). Such a process may be referred to as metabolic toxication. It should be recognized that whether or not metabolic toxication has practical significance depends on the quantity and potency of the metabolic product that is made available to the animal or biologic specimen

TABLE 4.1 Increased Toxicity Resulting from Metabolic Conversion

Compound	Product
Sulfanilamide	Acetylsulfanilamide
Ethylene glycol	Oxalic acid
Methanol	Formate
Fluoroacetate	Fluorocitrate
Parathion	Paraoxon
Tremorine	Oxytremorine
Tri-o-cresyl phosphate	Cyclic phosphate
Dimethyl nitroso amine	Diazomethane
Schradan	Schradan-N-oxide
Heptachlor	Heptachlor epoxide
Pyridine	n-Methyl pyridinium chloride
Chloral hydrate	Trichlorethanol chloride
Nitrobenzene	Nitrosobenzene, phenylhydroxylamine
Acetanilid	Analine
Pentavalent arsenicals	Trivalent arsenicals
Selenate	Selenite
2-Naphthylamine	2 Amino-l-naphthol
Codeine	Morphine
Phenylthiourea	Hydrogen sulfide

Note. Data from Schuster, L.: Metabolism of drugs and toxic substances. *Ann. Rev. Biochem.* **33:**590, 1964.

under consideration. It is apparent that metabolic toxication resulting from the conversion of Parathion to Paraoxon in an insect is significant; otherwise Parathion would be a most ineffective insecticide. In regard to conversion of sulfanilamide to acetyl sulfanilamide, this is a critical conjugation reaction in regard to lethal effect on bacteria, but is of little practical importance (except for changes in solubility leading to crystalluria) in regard to lethal toxicity in the average clinical case which is treated with sulfanilamide or similar therapeutic agents.

The effect of biotransformation of a compound may be of great significance in some examples but may be of no significance in other examples as far as the overall toxicity to the animals is concerned. An example in which the biotransformation process is of great significance is shown when a chemically unreactive compound is converted to highly reactive derivatives, where the derivatives are alkylating agents that are incorporated into macromolecules in the tissue cells. The enzymes that perform this conversion are in the mixed function oxidase system of the microsomes. The chemically reactive compound that is created may be only an intermediate in the total biotransformation reaction. For example, para-bromobenzene forms several derivatives in the liver. It is first converted to the active alkylating agent, bromobenzene epoxide, which undergoes rearrangement to form parabromophenol. These reactions are shown below.

In this example the epoxide is probably the principal compound that covalently binds with the macromolecules in the liver resulting in liver toxicity. An important concept resulting from the above example is that if the biotransformation process results in the formation of highly reactive derivatives such agents are capable of modifying vital macromolecules.

The microsomal oxidizing system has acquired added significance in toxicology because it is the basis of some popular theories about the mechanism of chemical-induced necrosis (i.e., death) of cells. One theory is that compounds that produce cell death selectively in specific species or organs and tissues within a given species do so because of the abundance in those tissues of the microsomal oxidizing system, and because intermediate reactive products capable of binding with essential proteins in the cell are formed by the oxidation of the parent compound. In fact, it is often possible to show a direct relationship between the severity of the tissue lesion and the amount of metabolite that is covalently bound in the damaged tissue. Also, by inhibiting the microsomal system, the tissue lesion is favorably influenced. Metabolic activation of a chemical resulting in tissue injury is the most probable mechanism responsible for local tissue damage occurring in only selected species as well as in only selected organs.

An example in which biotransformation of a compound to a more toxic agent has little significance in normal humans is the case of the metabolism of ethyl alcohol. The principal metabolism of ethyl alcohol does not involve the microsomal system. It involves conversion of ethanol to acetaldehyde by alcohol dehydrogenase (ADH) in the presence of nicotinamide adenine dinucleotide (NAD). The aldehyde is then converted to acetate. The acetate forms acetyl CoA which then enters the citric acid cycle. The end products are then carbon dioxide and water as follows:

$$Ethanol + NAD + ADH \rightarrow acetaldehyde + NADH$$
$$Acetaldehyde + aldehyde\ dehydrogenase \rightarrow acetate$$
$$Acetate + CoA \rightarrow acetyl\ CoA \rightarrow CO_2 + H_2O$$

In the human small amounts of acetaldehyde produce nausea, vomiting, headache, palpitation, and a fall in blood pressure. In the normal human, acetaldehyde never accumulates to any significant amount following ingestion of alcohol since it is rapidly converted to acetate. However, the enzyme system responsible for conversion of acetaldehyde to acetate can be blocked by administration of several compounds, among which is tetraethylthiouram disulfide; only when the aldehyde dehydrogenase enzyme is blocked does the ingestion of alcohol produce the characteristic symptoms of accumulation of acetaldehyde.

Whether or not toxicity occurs as a result of biotransformation to a more toxic substance is dependent on the affinity of the products of the reaction for receptors, the concentration of the product at the receptor sites, and the duration of its presence in the biologic system.

Inhibition of Biotransformation Mechanisms

Various circumstances can influence the level of the microsomal P450 enzyme system and thereby influence the toxicity of compounds that are dependent on this system for conversion to metabolites that are more or less toxic than the parent compound. It has been shown that even the diet can influence the level of the P450 system in experimental animals; that is, low-protein diets suppress P450 levels and associated enzyme activity.

The microsomal enzyme systems can be inhibited by several compounds in concentrations which by themselves have little definite pharmacologic activity. One of the first examples of a nonspecific microsomal enzyme inhibitor was SKF-525A (diethyl aminoethanol ester of diphenylpropyl acetic acid). This compound was initially investigated in 1954 and 1955 and was shown to increase the duration of a barbiturate-induced anesthesia, probably by directly combining with and inactivating the microsomal drug-metabolizing enzymes that are largely responsible for termination of the action of the barbiturate. The action of SKF-525A is not limited to an effect on barbiturate metabolism; rather, it has a general inhibitory action on many of the microsomal drug-metabolizing enzymes, and therefore may affect the metabolism of many xenobiotics normally metabolized by these enzymes.

When the product of metabolic transformation is of greater toxicity (metabolic toxication) than that of the parent compound, the inhibition of the metabolizing enzymes would be expected to protect the animal from toxicity resulting from metabolism of the parent compound. A good example is in regard to the liver lesions produced by large doses of the commonly used analgesic drug acetaminophen, which has been discussed previously in this chapter and is shown in Fig. 4.4. When animals are pre-treated with inhibitors of drug-metabolizing enzymes, the liver lesions are prevented from occurring. Such experiments initially suggested that the acetaminophen-induced hepatic necrosis is caused by a toxic metabolite rather than acetaminophen itself. However, this is not always the case; actual experiments with the phosphorothionates which are biotransformed to the more toxic O-analogs show that their toxicity is not affected by SKF-525A. This is because both the formation (metabolic toxication) and the hydrolysis (metabolic detoxication) of the O-analog are only partially blocked by SKF-525A; thus the two effects cancel each other. In contrast to this, in the case of procaine which is in part detoxified by microsomal esterases (metabolic detoxication), pretreatment of mice with SKF-525A decreases the LD_{50} of procaine from 188 to 79 mg/kg. In this case, the toxicity of procaine may be said to be increased by the pretreatment of the mice with SKF-525A. Since this effect of SKF-525A is the result of prolonging the metabolic conversion of procaine, it is a practical demonstration that the toxicity of a compound may be related to its duration of action in the organism, which is in turn related to the efficiency of the mechanisms involved in termination of action of the chemical in the organism. Other compounds that have the same action as SKF-525A are piperonyl butoxide and cobalt chloride.

Other factors also can be the cause of decreased microsomal enzyme activity. At least in rats, starvation for as little as 16 to 36 hr leads to the formation of an endogenous inhibitor of microsomal N-demethylation. There is also ample evidence that the livers of newborn as well as immature animals are deficient in the microsomal drug metabolizing enzymes. There-fore, these as well as various as yet undetermined factors may alter the activity of the microsomal enzymes and may account in part for variations in toxicity within members of a species.

Inhibition of microsomal as well as nonmicrosomal enzyme systems is occasionally involved in drug interactions that result in toxicity. Many drugs produce their therapeutic effects by inhibition of specific enzyme systems; when a second drug is given in several doses to the patient, if that second drug is dependent on the affected enzyme system for termination of its presence in the body, the second drug will accumulate in the patient with each subsequent dose. For example, allopurinol is a xanthine oxidase inhibitor that reduces the synthesis of uric acid in some species of animals and in man. It is used in the treatment of gout and other clinical states associated with increased levels of uric acid. Other drugs such as 6-mercaptopurine (an antileukemic drug) and azathioprine (an immunosuppressant drug) are normally inactivated by xanthine oxidase. Concomitant repeated administration of allopurinol with 6-mercaptopurine or azathioprine will increase the plasma levels of the latter drugs, and because of the profound suppressant effect of these drugs on the tissue responsible for the formation of blood cells, such interactions can be fatal.

It is practically impossible to determine the effects of all possible drug or chemical combinations. If the mechanism of termination of biologic action of any agent is via an enzyme system, then it is highly probable that other agents which influence the enzyme will alter the toxicity of the first compound. Therefore whenever a drug is a known enzyme inhibitor, toxicity tests should be conducted in combination with other drugs that are dependent on that enzyme system for their inactivation.

Induction of Biotransformation Mechanisms

The total quantity of microsomal drug-metabolizing enzymes can be increased in humans and in higher animals by prior administration of a large variety of chemical substances. Such substances include the anesthetics, such as nitrous oxide, ether, and chloroform; the sedatives, such as barbiturates and urethane; analgesics, such as glutethimide and phenylbutazone; the hypoglycemic agents, such as tolbutamide and carbutamide; and the insecticides, the particularly effective ones being chlordane, DDT, hexachlorocyclohexane, dieldrin, aldrin, and heptachlor.

Induction of enzyme activity usually involves repeated exposure to the inducing chemical. It is usually temporary and lasts from 2 to 4 weeks following the administration of the inducing chemical. When phenobarbital is injected daily for 5 days in anesthetic doses in the dog, the duration and half-life of the drug in the blood are shortened. Four weeks later the half-life of the drug in the blood as well as the duration of anesthesia has returned to normal. Currently it is not clear what the duration of enhanced microsomal enzyme activity may be following repeated daily exposure to organochlorine pesticides which may exist as residues on food consumed by humans or animals.

The phenomenon of chemical-induced enhancement of the activity of enzyme systems that are responsible for their own degradation apparently results in an increased rate of metabolic transformation of the compound. Since metabolic transformation has been shown to result in the formation of more or less toxic products as compared to the parent compound, enzyme induction may be protective to the animal (when detoxication is involved) or detrimental to the animal (when toxication is involved). The induction of enzymes by the administration of chemicals basically represents a mechanism of adaptation by the animal to repeated assault by foreign chemicals. This type of adaptation does not represent a true tolerance, which has been defined as a modified response of the receptor.

It is now recognized that the microsomal mixed-function oxidases of the endoplasmic reticulum are initially inhibited by high concentrations of those compounds which are normally used as substrates for the system. Good examples of such substrates are the barbiturate drugs and the halogenated hydrocarbon pesticides. The initial inhibition of the enzymes by these compounds is believed to be an important step in the subsequent induction of the same enzymes, that is, substrates that are slowly metabolized act as inhibitors and initiate a feedback mechanism that calls for additional *de novo* synthesis of the oxidase proteins. Furthermore, the nature of the induced enzyme is influenced by the type of inducer involved. For example the carcinogenic polycyclic aromatic hydrocarbons such as benzo(a)pyrene and 3-methyl-cholanthrene are slow inducers which initially produce a conformational change in cytochrome P450, converting it to P448; the new enzyme is synthesized *de novo* as cytochrome P448. Currently cytochrome P450 has become recognized as the terminal oxidase that is induced by many drugs and pesticides, whereas cytochrome P448 is induced by recognized carcinogenic agents. Furthermore, cytochrome P450 may actually be destroyed by reacting irreversibly with some highly reactive intermediate radicals that it is responsible for producing. For example, many organic sulfur-containing compounds are desulfated and converted to their oxygen analogs by the microsomal mixed function oxidases; the sulfur which is released forms a stable complex with cytochrome P450, thereby inactivating it.

An important consequence of enzyme induction is that when the microsomal enzymes are induced by one compound and a second compound is then introduced into the animal, if the second compound is metabolized by the same enzyme system its metabolism will also be altered. In this manner the toxicity of the second compound will be either increased or decreased depending on the products of the biotransformation reaction. In chronic drug therapy indirect drug interactions due to this mechanism can seriously alter the therapeutic efficiency and toxicity of other drugs that may be concomitantly administered to the patient.

The foregoing discussion of metabolic transformation mechanisms suggests at least two important possibilities by which chemical-induced toxicity can be altered. The first is that toxicity of a given compound can be distinctly different within members of a species or between species if the suitable enzymatic systems between the test organisms are not identical. The second is that prior exposure to a chemical can alter the toxicity of the same chemical and other chemicals to which the biologic specimen may be exposed on a subsequent occasion.

CHAPTER **5**

Influence of Route
of Administration on
Systemic Toxicity

Under normal day-to-day conditions humans, as well as essentially all mammals, are exposed to chemicals in the air, in food, and in drinking water. In addition, humans are exposed to a wide variety of agents which are applied to the skin for cleansing or cosmetic reasons or ingested for therapeutic or recreational purposes. The chemical and physical properties of each compound largely determine the route by which exposure can occur. For example, although solids can be suspended in the air as "dusts," vapors and gases would be the most common, readily available agents for inhalation via the respiratory route. Xenobiotic materials which are dissolved or suspended in water would be ingested by the oral route, in which case absorption could take place through the gastrointestinal tract. Thus the percutaneous (or dermal), the oral (or gastrointestinal) route, and the inhalation (or respiratory route) are the common routes by which xenobiotic agents gain access to biologic systems in animals. However, under experimental conditions in the laboratory in which the toxicologist wishes to produce and study harmful effects of chemicals, additional routes of exposure are commonly used. These routes involve a group of techniques by which agents are injected into various body compartments. In this case the common routes of exposure involve injection directly into the blood (intravenous route), into the abdominal fluid (intraperitoneal route), beneath the skin (subcutaneous route), into the spinal subarachnoid fluid (intrathecal route), or into a muscle (intramuscular route). The route of administration of an agent determines the barriers that the agent will encounter in regard to absorption, distribution, and biotransformation. Although the route of administration has little to do with the qualitative nature of the toxicity of a compound, it can greatly influence the quantitative toxicologic response to an agent; that is, it can alter the slope and position of the dose–response curve.

PERCUTANEOUS ROUTE

The skin of humans is fundamentally a modified membrane comparable to the mucous membranes of the mouth and gastrointestinal and respiratory tracts. It acts as a barrier to the transfer of xenobiotics in a manner similar to the other mucous membranes. It consists of two layers, an outer epithelial layer known as the epidermis and an underlying connective tissue layer known as the dermis (or corium). The epidermis consists of continuous multilayers of cells pierced only by the orifices of the hair follicles and sweat gland ducts. The sweat glands and hair follicles are embedded in the dermis. The sebaceous glands generally open into the hair follicles. The effectiveness of the skin as a barrier to the transfer of xenobiotics varies considerably at different sites on the body and for different xenobiotics.

When chemicals are applied to the skin toxicity may be manifested at the site of application and the agent may be translocated through the skin, resulting in adverse systemic effects. In general it is clear that the amount of any compound that passes through the skin is dependent on the applied dose, the time over which the agent is in contact with the skin, the concentration involved, and the location as well as the surface area involved. In addition a compound may be exposed to multiple enzymes in the skin that may transform the initial compound into products having different chemical properties and toxicities. When these factors are determined for a given agent dermal absorption rates can be predicted. This has been very successfully utilized in the drug industry to administer such drugs as nitroglycerin and scopolamine which are incorporated in patches that are applied to the skin. A single patch is designed to supply the drug in therapeutic amounts slowly and uniformly over a 24-hr period.

The barrier properties of whole skin vary with the site of application and with the properties of the chemical which is applied, both in the same species and in different species. Pig skin appears to have a higher diffusion rate for water than does rat or guinea pig skin. As an example Table 5.1 indicates the species variation in percutaneous toxicities of two organic phosphates. Furthermore, the integrity of the skin barrier can be altered by application of chemicals which specifically produce a breakdown in the surface layer, an example being formic acid. Methyl and ethyl alcohol, hexane, and acetone applied to the skin and washed off may be used as solvents for the normal lipids in the skin resulting in a moderate change in permeability. A marked change in skin permeability can be produced by application of chloroform–methanol (2:1) mixture. The normal rat skin can be penetrated by a variety of chemical agents. Simple organic amines such as propyl, butyl, and pentyl amines have been shown to penetrate rat skin at a rate that increases linearly with concentration. These amines penetrate the skin only in an unchanged state, so that below the isoelectric point where the amines exist as cations, penetration through the skin is poor.

The physicochemical properties of the substance under consideration are the principal determining factors with respect to percutaneous absorption of the compound. In general, it may be thought that gases penetrate quite freely through the epidermal tissues, liquids less freely, and solids which are insoluble in water or lipids probably are incapable of penetrating to a significant degree. Solids that are soluble in the secretions of the skin may dissolve in the secretions to a variable extent and thereby be put into solution. Penetration of materials through the skin is time-dependent, and this can be demonstrated by the application of occlusive bandages to prevent loss of the material from the site of application.

TABLE 5.1 **Relative Percutaneous Toxicities of Two Organophosphorus Compounds Tested in Eight Animal Species[a]**

Species	Compound A[b]	Compound B[b]	B/A
Rabbit	1.0	5.0	5.0
Pig	10.0	80.0	8.0
Dog	1.9	10.8	5.7
Monkey	4.4	~13.0	~3.0
Goat	~3.0	~4.0	~1.3
Cat	0.9	2.4	2.7
Mouse	6.0	~9.2	~1.5
Rat	17.0	20.0	1.2

[a] Data from McCreesh, A. H.: Percutaneous toxicity. *Toxicol. Appl. Pharmacol.* **7**:20, 1965.
[b] All values expressed as ratio of the LD_{50} of that compound to the rabbit LD_{50} of Compound A.

Although it is not clear to what extent lipid solubility of the compound is important, it is apparent that both water and lipid solubility influence percutaneous penetration of a compound. The insecticide DDT is considerably more soluble in lipids than it is in water. It is also more poorly absorbed from the skin than it is from the gastrointestinal tract. The comparative LD_{50}'s for DDT in rats for the oral and dermal routes of administration are 118 and 2510 mg/kg, respectively. In contrast to this the insecticide Isolan is quite soluble in water, is well absorbed from the skin, and is more toxic by dermal than by oral administration to rats. Prominent among the lipid-soluble compounds readily absorbed into the skin are phenol and phenolic derivatives; hormones such as estrogen, progesterone, testosterone, and desoxycorticosterone; vitamins D and K; and organic bases such as strychnine and nicotine. As far as polarity is concerned, it appears that nonpolar compounds pass through the skin more readily than ionic materials, but not exclusively so. Salts of some alkaloids may pass freely through the skin.

A variety of factors such as pH, extent of ionization, molecular size, and water and lipid solubility are all involved with the transfer of chemicals through the skin. Local factors such as temperature and blood flow to the site will influence the rate of absorption and therefore the percutaneous toxicity of potent chemicals.

INHALATION ROUTE

Exposure to chemicals in the atmosphere is accomplished by unavoidable inhalation of such agents unless devices are used to remove the atmospheric contaminants before they enter the respiratory tract. However, in order for any particular chemical contaminant to reach the alveoli of the lungs, it must be a gas, a vapor, or of sufficiently proper particulate size so that it is not removed in the airway to the lungs. Although some atmospheric contaminants present little more than a nuisance, others are capable of inducing local as well as systemic toxicity. The actual and potential hazards associated with exposure to chemicals via the respiratory tract are particularly evident in regard to industrial working environments and in regard to pollution of atmospheres in urban areas of high-density human populations.

Because of the widespread use of a large number of chemicals in industrial working environments, it is not surprising that the atmosphere in which people work is more or less contaminated with a variety of such chemicals. It has therefore become necessary to establish some standards regarding the limits of contamination of the atmosphere which would be considered safe. The data necessary to establish a maximum safe concentration of a chemical in the atmosphere for humans who are exposed over an 8-hr working day are only rarely obtainable. Those values that are available for specific chemicals represent estimations based on information obtained by experience in industry and by experiments on humans and animals.

The American National Standards Institutes (ANSI) initially recognized and developed some guidelines for use in industrial toxicology regarding safe exposure concentrations to some chemicals in the work environment. These were soon adopted by the American Conference of Governmental Industrial Hygienists (ACGIH) who initially published what are now recognized as Threshold Limit Values (TLVs). Initially a TLV was a maximum concentration of an agent in air that was believed to be "safe" for exposure in the working environment for a lifetime. In the United States in 1970 the National Institute of Occupational Safety and Health (NIOSH) Act emphasized the need for some regulatory standard consensus of opinion regarding safe levels for inhalation exposure to chemical contaminants in the workplace. NIOSH adapted TLVs as the legal permissible levels (PELs) and issued criterion documents for many of the common industrial air contaminants. Actually, TLVs are reviewed annually by the ACGIH committee but have no legal status, whereas PELs have legal status in the United States and can be changed only by legislative action. More recently the degree of sophistication of TLVs has greatly improved so that ACGIH now lists TLVs as time-weighted averages (TWAs) and may include short-term exposure limits (STELs) and a ceiling concentration limit (TLV-C). STELs represent a maximum concentration limit for a period of not more than 15 min. As the term indicates, TWAs are the average allowable values over an 8-hr period of time and take into account periodic exposures above and below the average. Although PELs have legal status they have no more scientific validity than TLVs. For details on this subject the reader is referred to the National Research Council publication in 1983 on "Risk Assessment in the Federal Government: Managing the Process" and in 1994 on "Science and Judgment in the Risk Assessment."

Inhalation of toxicants is an unintentional means or route of exposure to xenobiotics whether it involves an industrial or urban environment. Consequently it has become a subject of considerable public interest and federal regulatory action. The current extremely conservative policies of the federal regulation agencies in the United States have resulted in questions about the ability of both science and the regulatory agencies to accurately evaluate the threat of harmful effects from inhalation of toxicants. This book has stressed that from a scientific perspective toxicity is a graded effect, and that there is no sharp line that distinguishes between harmful and safe doses for any xenobiotic agent. Further consideration of this subject is beyond the scope of this book, which acknowledges the respiratory route as a principal route of exposure to gases, vapors, and even particulate materials. This has resulted in a vast body of literature with its own terminology, as well as controversial regulatory legislation.

TLVs serve a useful purpose in that they represent a gross classification of the relative harmfulness or safeness of a large variety of compounds that become atmospheric pollutants in industry. Their use for any other purpose is grossly erroneous, if one accepts the concept that all harmful effects of chemicals are graded responses that are dose-dependent and that there is no exact concentration of a chemical above which that chemical is harmful or below which it is safe. The only way in which any value which represents a safe value for human exposure can be established is through extensive experience; even then, such a value would not represent a "limit," but would only represent an estimated safe level for exposure. The 6th edition (1991) of *TLV Documentation for Chemical Substances in the Work Environment* lists data for approximately 700 compounds. Some examples of the TLVs listed are given in Table 5.2.

ORAL ROUTE

The oral route is probably the third most common means by which a chemical enters the body. The gastrointestinal tract in the experimental

TABLE 5.2 A Selected List of Threshold Limit Values

Compound	TLV–TWA (ppm)[a]	TLV–STEL (ppm)[a]
Bis (chloromethyl) ether	0.001	—
Toluene-2,4-diisocyanate	0.005	0.02
Methyl isocyanate	0.02	—
Nickel carbonyl (as Ni)	0.05	—
Acrolein	0.1	0.3
Chloropicrin	10	—
Hexane	50	—
Turpentine	100	—
Methyl alcohol	200	250
Gasoline	300	500
Acetone	750	1000
Butane	800	—
Ethyl alcohol	1000	—
Carbon dioxide	5000	30,000

Note. From *Documentation of TLVs and Biological Exposure Indices,* 6th ed., American Association of Governmental Industrial Hygienists, 1991.

[a] Parts of vapor or gas per million parts of air volume at 25°C and 760 mm Hg.

animal may be viewed as a tube going through the body, starting at the mouth and ending at the anus. Although it is within the body, its contents are essentially exterior to the body fluids. Therefore, chemicals in the gastrointestinal tract can produce an effect only on the surface of the mucosal cells that line the tract, unless absorption from the gastrointestinal tract takes place. Caustic or primary irritant agents, such as strong alkalis and acids or the phenols, in adequate concentration can result in a direct necrotizing effect on the mucosa of the tract. Most orally administered chemicals can otherwise have a systemic effect on the organism only after absorption has occurred from the mouth or the gastrointestinal tract.

Although alcohol, nitroglycerin, and even several of the steroid drugs can be absorbed directly through oral mucosa, they must be retained in the mouth for a suitable time interval if any significant absorption is to take place. Under ordinary conditions, chemicals or even foods remain in the mouth and esophagus for too short a time to permit any significant degree of absorption. Rather, the first site from which orally administered chemicals can be effectively translocated is the stomach (or the rumen in those species that have such organs).

The effect of the special condition of pH in the stomach and the influence of pH on the ionization of the weak organic acids and bases have been described in the previous chapter. In the stomach the chemical comes in contact with preexisting stomach contents (such as food particles and gastric mucin) and secretions (such as pepsin, renin, and gastric lipase) in addition to hydrochloric acid. If the chemical was to be absorbed, react with, or act as a substrate for any of these components of the gastric contents, the amount of free chemical would be altered, thereby leading to an altered absorption rate of the agent. Products of reactions that take place in the stomach may be more or less readily translocated or more or less toxic than the parent compound. As the orally ingested compound is carried from the stomach into the intestine, the pH is again shifted and the chemical is mixed further with additional agents such as the food residues, bile, and the additional enzymes in the pancreatic juice.

The toxicity of orally administered chemicals may vary with the frequency with which they are given, and with the conditions under which they are given (that is, whether they are mixed with food or given on an empty stomach). Studies regarding two examples show that the toxicity of a drug given by oral gavage (introduction via stomach tube) may be considerably different from the same drug administered by admixture in the diet. The drugs used were Dimethline (a respiratory stimulant) and Dixyrazine (a phenothiazine type drug used as a tranquilizing agent). Dimethline possessed much greater lethal toxicity when administered by gavage than when given in the diet, whereas Dixyrazine showed the opposite behavior. When Dimethline was administered to fasted rats by gavage, the LD_{50} was found to be about 12 mg/kg. When the rats remained unfasted, this value was 30 mg/kg. With repeated daily gavage, 5 mg/kg was tolerated, whereas 10 mg/kg was fatal. The symptomology was the same in all cases. When the same drug was administered in the diet, the rats tolerated 100 mg/kg, which is 10 times the lethal gavage level. Further studies indicated that the drug remained unchanged chemically in the diet, that acute toxicity was less in unfasted than in fasted rats, that by employing divided dose procedures the normally acute lethal dose could be tolerated for several weeks. Similar studies performed with Dixyrazine indicated that it was appreciably more toxic when administered in the diet than when given by gavage. In this case, analysis of the test diet showed that 60% of the chemical underwent degradation when mixed with the diet, and it appeared that the products of degradation were more toxic than the original material.

An example in which oral toxicity is greater when the substance is administered in the feed than when given by stomach tube or gavage is the case of griseofulvin; administered by the oral route, this is normally a substance of low toxicity. When this substance is added to the feed of mice, it leads to pathologic changes in the liver, although such changes are not encountered in rats, guinea pigs, or rabbits. In mice, the addition of griseofulvin to the diet resulted in changes in the biliary tract in 10 to 12 days and tumors of the liver at 140 days. When an equivalent dose of griseofulvin was given as a single dose by stomach tube, only slight liver damage was observed even after a period of 122 days. When the single daily dose was divided into nine fractional doses given at 1-hr intervals during each day, microscopic changes in the liver did occur on the third and fourth day. Therefore, it would appear that if the objective of the test is to obtain toxicity, it would be preferable to administer the griseofulvin in the feed rather than by gavage.

Following oral administration of a compound to animals, absorption of the agent from the gut necessarily involves translocation of the agent either to the lymphatic system or to the portal circulation. Those agents that appear in the portal circulation are carried directly to the liver. A large number of foreign compounds that appear in the blood following their absorption from the gut are known to be excreted by the liver into the bile. Thus, a cycle involving translocation of the chemical from the intestine to the liver and to the bile and back to the intestine is established. This cycle is referred to as the *enterohepatic circulation.* Some compounds simply diffuse from the blood into the bile, whereas others are actively excreted into the bile. For example, the bile salts and Bromsulphalein appear in the bile in concentrations from 10 to 1000 times greater than the concentrations of the compound in the blood, whereas compounds such as glucose appear in the bile in a concentration less than that which is present in blood.

Furthermore, the liver may biotransform or conjugate a chemical, for example with glucuronide or sulfate, and excrete the conjugate into the bile where the metabolite is then carried to the intestine, and reabsorbed back into the portal circulation. The drugs madribon and chloramphenicol appear to be actively excreted in the bile as the glucuronides and the conjugates are then hydrolyzed in the gut to yield the initial form of the drugs, which are in turn absorbed again into the portal circulation and thereby enter the cycle of the enterohepatic system. Studies of the enterohepatic circulation of a series of nitro- and hydroxybenzoic acids in rats and have shown that both molecular size and degree of conjugation influence biliary excretion of the compounds. Several of the chlorinated hydrocarbon insecticides are also known to undergo enterohepatic circulation in various laboratory animals. Prominent among such insecticides are DDT (2,2-bis [parachlorphenyl] 1,1,1-trichlorethane), aldrin, dieldrin, and methoxychlor. The liver appears to be an important site for biotransformation of DDT to DDE (2,2-bis [parachlorphenyl] 1,1-dichlorethane) and other metabolites, a process which leads to the excretion of DDE in the bile. This mechanism is the principal source for the appearance of DDT metabolites in the feces. Surgical obstruction of the biliary duct in rats that are given isotope-tagged DDT leads to increased excretion of the isotope in the urine, indicating that the enterohepatic circulation also consitutes a mechanism of termination of action of this compound.

Oral administration of chemicals that are rapidly absorbed from the gastrointestinal tract would theoretically expose the liver to concentrations of the agent that would not be obtained by other routes of administration. Furthermore, if a compound entered the enterohepatic cycle, at least a portion of the compound would be localized in the organs involved in the cycle. Compounds that are known to be toxic to the liver would be expected to be more toxic following oral administration on repeated occasions, whereas their administration by other routes may be less hazardous. An example of this is in the use of thiopental. This drug is a short-acting thiobarbiturate which is commonly administered intravenously to produce anesthesia. Intravenous use of this drug has not been noted for its hepatotoxicity. The compound is readily absorbed from the stomach and intestine, but repeated use of the compound by the oral route of administration in experimental animals is likely to produce degenerative changes in the liver; therefore, its use by the oral route is not recommended in humans.

PARENTERAL ROUTES

Introduction of chemicals into the organism by means of injection of the chemical from a syringe through a hollow needle at specific sites in the animal is a common procedure used in the administration of drugs. By this means, the natural body orifices are bypassed and specific amounts, or doses, of chemicals may be introduced into the animal. These routes of administration are collectively called the parenteral routes of administration of chemicals. They consist of administration of chemicals by injection into the skin (intrademal), beneath the skin (subcutaneous), in the muscle (intramuscular), into the blood of the veins (intravenous), or into the spinal fluid (intrathecal). Specific agents may on infrequent occasions be administered into the blood in the arteries (intraarterial), into tumors, or into the chest fluid (intrapleural). In laboratory animals, the injection of chemicals into the abdominal fluid (intraperitoneal) is a very common procedure, whereas this is only done in humans on extremely rare occasions. In the laboratory, it is even possible to inject solutions into single cells (intracellular) by use of micropipettes.

It is apparent that the most rapid means of achieving a high concentration of a chemical within a given tissue is to introduce the chemical directly into that tissue. Whereas intravenous administration of a chemical bypasses the biologic barriers presented by the normal body surface or orifices, other parenteral routes may impose additional barriers to translocation of the chemical. In the latter case, the chemical remains at its site of deposition until absorption or diffusion carries it to the sites in the animal where it can be chemically modified or excreted. Therefore, except for a local action at the site of injection, parenteral administration of chemicals still necessitates translocation of the agent in the organism if the chemical is to reach distant specific receptor sites.

Lethal toxicity of a chemical may be dependent or variously independent of the route of parenteral administration. Examples of compounds for which the LD_{50} is dependent and independent of the route of administration are given in Table 5.3. In general, it may be assumed that the intensity of the toxicity of a compound will be different following different parenteral routes of administration if the rate at which translocation of the compound takes place is influenced by the injection route. For example, if the rate of absorption from the site of administration is less than the rate of excretion (or termination of action of the compound), there will be little opportunity for accumulation of a biologically effective systemic concentration of the compound. In contrast to this, if the rate of termination of action of the compound is less than the rate of absorption from the site of administration, it would be reasonable to expect the compound to achieve systemically effective concentrations.

These facts are utilized in the development of drug formulations when it is desired to achieve a constant systemic concentration of a drug over a period of time. This condition is practically accomplished by developing a

TABLE 5.3 Effects of Administration of Compounds in Which Lethal Toxicity Is Independent (Isoniazid), Partially Dependent (DFP and Pentobarbital), and Completely Dependent (Procaine) on Route of Administration

Route of administration	Procaine[a] (mouse) LD$_{50}$ (mg/kg)	Ratio (X/IV)	Isoniazid[a] (mouse) LD$_{50}$ (mg/kg)	Ratio (X/IV)	DFP[b] (rabbit) LD$_{50}$ (mg/kg)	Ratio (X/IV)	Pentobarbital[a] (mouse) LD$_{50}$ (mg/kg)	Ratio (X/IV)
Intravenous	45	1	153	1.0	0.34	1.0	80	1.0
Intraperitoneal	230	5	132	0.9	1.00	2.9	130	1.6
Intramuscular	630	14	140	0.9	0.85	2.5	124	1.5
Subcutaneous	800	18	160	1.0	1.00	2.9	130[c]	1.6
Oral	500	11	142	0.9	4 to 9	11.7 to 26.5	280	3.5

[a] Data from Barnes, C. D., and Eltherington, L. G.: *Drug Dosage in Laboratory Animals.* University of California Press, Berkeley, CA, 1964.
[b] DFP, diisopropylfluorophosphate. Data from Spector, W. S. (Ed.): *Handbook of Toxicology,* Vol. I, Acute Toxicities. W. B. Saunders, Philadelphia, 1956.
[c] Personal data from author's laboratory.

formulation of a drug which only permits slow liberation and absorption of the drug following intramuscular or subcutaneous administration of the preparation. A good example of such a preparation is procaine penicillin as compared to penicillin. The former preparation permits slow absorption of the penicillin from intramuscular sites as compared to the latter preparation which is rapidly absorbed. The natural counterpart of this mechanism is the buffering effect involved in adsorption of drugs to plasma protein, thereby limiting the quantity of free active drug in the circulation regardless of the route of administration of the drug.

Intraperitoneal injection of chemicals represents a selective site of administration in which an absorbable chemical will first be translocated to the liver via the portal circulation. This is possible because the major venous blood circulation from the abdominal contents of mammals is effected via the portal circulation. Therefore, an intraperitoneally administered compound is subjected to the special metabolic transformation mechanisms existent in the liver, as well as to the possibility of excretion of the compound in the bile before it gains access to the remainder of the animal. A hypothetical compound which is selectively toxic to any system in the animal other than the liver, and which is detoxified in the liver, would be expected to have a greater toxicity following subcutaneous or intravenous administration than following intraperitoneal administration. An example of such a compound is the organic phosphate Soman (methyl pinacolyl phosphonofluoridate) for which the LD_{50}'s in the mouse are, respectively, 0.165 and 0.425 mg/kg by the subcutaneous and intraperitoneal routes of administration. The LD_{50} values of compounds that were not biotransformed or excreted into the bile would not be expected to be different by the intraperitoneal as compared to the subcutaneous or intravenous routes of administration unless other factors, such as differences in absorption from the three sites, were involved. Therefore, it is possible to predict some information regarding translocation, deposition, inactivation, or site of excretion from comparative evaluation of LD_{50}'s of a given compound which are determined by various routes of administration.

The specific biologic barriers that are effective in blocking translocation of compounds in an animal effectively protect certain tissues from exposure to a large number of foreign chemicals, although the chemicals may be present in the blood of the animal. An excellent example of this is the blood–brain barrier in mammals, which inhibits translocation of quaternized nitrogen-containing compounds from the blood to the central nervous system. Intrathecally administered chemicals bypass the blood–brain barrier, thereby permitting the brain to receive concentrations of the agent that could not be obtained by any other route of administration. Certain antibiotic drugs are therefore administered by direct intrathecal injection for treatment of infections of the brain and spinal cord. Administration of proper volumes as well as amounts of local anesthetic agents, such as procaine or pontocaine solutions, by intrathecal administration produce spinal anesthesia, whereas the same compounds are ineffective as spinal anesthetic agents when given by other routes. Thus, toxicity following intrathecal administration varies as compared to other routes of administration depending upon the site of action of the agent under consideration and on the barriers to translocation of the compound.

The intravenous route of administration of liquids and the inhalation route for gases and vapors achieve rapid systemic distribution of the compound throughout the animal. The compound reaches all organs of the animal in periods of time limited only by the time required for the blood to circulate and the time necessary for translocation of the compound from the capillaries to the extracellular fluid. Compounds with rapid biologic action therefore generally show greater toxicity following intravenous administration than when they are given by other parenteral routes.

The foregoing discussion has been oriented toward the influence of the various routes of administration of chemicals on toxicity in the species of animals commonly utilized in the toxicology laboratory or in man. Comparable variations in routes of administration are adapted to other species, such as fish, birds, or insects, but are uncommon except for specific laboratory investigational work. The usual route of administration of chemicals to these latter species involves exposure via the environment of the species. Comparisons of toxicities between species of animals by similar routes of administration for various foreign chemicals frequently shed light on mechanisms of action, mechanisms of biotransformation, and mechanisms of excretion of chemicals of interest in toxicology.

CHAPTER **6**

Genetic Factors That Influence Toxicity

In most modern toxicology texts the subject of "Genetic Toxicology" deals entirely with the interaction of chemical agents with the hereditary mechanism. In this context Genetic Toxicology is a new specialty that has received recognition only during the past 30 years, and it is concerned with the demonstration of chemical-induced genetic damage. The discipline has developed both animal and clinical laboratory test methods to detect mutants as well as the mutations that they produce. These methods are described in Chapter 13. Chemical-induced mutagenicity is unique in toxicology because it can lead to acute toxicity in contemporary generations as well as in the subsequent offspring of affected subjects.

In this chapter the subject of Genetic Toxicology will be presented in a broader context; that is, it will consider not only chemicals acting as mutagens that damage the hereditary system alone, but also effects of variations in the "normal" genetic code as a cause of toxicity when man is exposed to other nonmutagenic xenobiotic chemicals.

THE GENETIC MECHANISM

The morphologic and biochemical makeup of biologic systems is determined by the heredity of the individual members. The basic units of inheritance are the genes, which are submicroscopic entities located at various areas on the chromosomes. Various species of animals possess various numbers of such gene-containing chromosomes which always exist in pairs (Fig. 6.1). Humans, for example, have 23 pairs of chromosomes. Each member of a pair is an autosome; therefore the human has 44 autosomes plus two sex chromosomes. In the female, each of the two sex chromosomes possess the "X" or sex-determining gene. In the male, one of the sex chromosomes contains the "X" gene and the other chromosome contains the "Y" gene. Thus, females possess the "XX" chromosomes and males

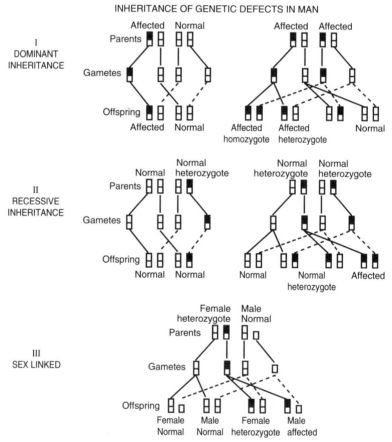

FIGURE 6.1 According to Hsia, D. Y., *Inborn Errors of Metabolism,* Year Book of Medical Publishers, Chicago, 1959, pp. 19–23. Examples consist of heterozygous state of the abnormality in which the paired chromosomes contain one normal gene (⊟) and one abnormal gene (▮).

possess the "XY" chromosomes. Those genes that are located at the same points on paired chromosomes are known as alleles.

A specific single gene or many genes may be responsible for a specific trait of the individual. If many genes are involved, the condition of polygenic inheritance for the specific trait is said to exist. Abnormalities that manifest themselves as altered morphology or altered ability to direct the synthesis of proteins originate as mutations. Since the normal is only apparent when a mutation occurs, a mutation (altered gene) may involve the ability of the progeny to carry on a vital function and such progeny would not survive. However, a mutation that affects the genetic template for the formation of a nonvital enzyme system may permit the progeny to survive, and may be manifested by the ability of the organism to produce either a deficient enzyme or a completely inactive enzyme. Such a genetically induced deficiency may go undetected until the deficient system is suitably challenged.

Drugs and chemicals represent possible challenging agents for the determination of the existence of certain enzymes within the body if these enzymes are involved in metabolic alteration of the drug or chemical. The origin of such mutations is not understood, although there is some evidence that a mutation can be induced by exposure of the reproductive cells to high-energy radiation or to formaldehyde or nitrogen mustard. The mutated gene may be dominant or recessive with respect to its ability to result in a manifested abnormality in the biologic organism. Figure 6.1 depicts the possible conditions that can exist when a single abnormal gene is considered in regard to inheritance of disease in man. Such concepts may be applicable to deficient enzyme systems that may be involved in metabolic transformation of chemicals in the intact biologic specimen. It is estimated that humans have at least 50,000 expressed genes; currently, some information is available for about 5000, and about 1900 have been mapped in terms of their chromosomal location. For information on the current status of Mendelian inheritance in man the reader is referred to McCusick, V. A., *Mendelian Inheritance in Man: Catalogs of Autosomal Dominant, Autosomal Recessive, and X-Linked Phenotypes,* Johns Hopkins Press, 1992.

CHEMICALS AS MUTAGENS

The evaluation of thousands of chemicals in the laboratory for their ability to produce damage to DNA has demonstrated that many agents possess this capability. Furthermore, it is generally recognized that it is highly probable that many carcinogens are mutagens and that many but not all mutagens are carcinogens. In addition, both of these classes of toxicity can be induced in cells which subsequently can undergo repair to normal. The recent human genome project to define the amino acid sequence of the genetic code has helped to increase the total body of knowledge about the genetic basis of human disease.

Currently it is believed that mutations of any cell type (somatic or germ) can be produced by some xenobiotic chemicals. Such mutations are subject to repair (removal of the damage) and may not result in permanent changes in the genetic code. Mutations in somatic cells that are lethal to the cell (such as those that are produced by cancer chemotherapeutic agents) are very useful as a therapeutic approach to the treatment of cancer. Nonlethal mutations in germ cells which do not undergo repair present the possibility of transfer to subsequent generations. Only in the past few years have the techniques in molecular biology become available to supply data for study by epidemiologic methods in humans. Consequently, when the simple, commonly encountered xenobiotic agent ethylene oxide was demonstrated in 1990 to produce genetic changes in male mouse germ cells, it supplied an impetus to evaluate the germinal changes (in terms of risk to humans) associated with occupational and environmental exposure to the compound.

Basically, current knowledge from animal and cellular experiments demonstrates that DNA of somatic and germ cells can be damaged by a variety of xenobiotic agents and that chromosomal and point mutations result from replication by the damaged template. To date, there are no conclusive examples of inheritable xenobiotic-induced disease in humans. Considerable effort is directed toward a better understanding of the risk involved when humans are exposed to "mutagenic" agents. In constrast all chemical-induced carcinogenic agents that have been demonstrated in man have also been demonstrated in animals.

PRINCIPLES OF GENETIC-INDUCED CHEMICAL TOXICITY

Termination of biologic action of chemicals in an organism is accomplished by excretion, by metabolic transformation processes, or by deposition mechanisms. Of the three processes, only excretion permanently removes the chemical from the body so that it can no longer produce a biologic effect. In contrast to this, metabolic transformation of a compound may lead to the formation of a more or less potent toxicant.

In cases in which the metabolic transformation process would convert the chemical to a *more* toxic compound, theoretically it would be better for the organism to have a deficiency of the enzyme involved, to ensure that *less* of the more toxic compound would be produced. In cases in which the metabolic transformation process would convert the chemical to a *less* toxic compound, a deficiency of the enzyme would be detrimental, because the organism then would not be able to remove the chemical by metabolic transformation, but would have to rely on other processes.

Since the enzymes involved in metabolic transformation of chemicals exist according to the genetic templates characteristic of each member of a population of organisms, genetic defects in members of a species may result in a deficiency or complete lack of certain enzymes. Such genetic defects within members of a species have been shown to be responsible for some specific types of toxicities from chemical agents. These forms of toxicity appear in the affected genotypes, and can be shown to occur at the frequencies stipulated by the laws of genetics. Genetically controlled deviations in individuals within a population therefore may be the reason certain "idiosyncratic" toxicities occur in a few members of a supposedly homogeneous population. Genetic deviations also represent one mechanism involved in biologic variation as it is manifested in relation to chemicals. The study of the genetically controlled factors that influence the pharmacologic actions of drugs has been termed "pharmacogenetics," but the usual example in pharmacogenetics involves examples of toxic effects of drugs as they are seen in relatively small numbers of a total population.

DISCOVERY AND CLASSIFICATION OF GENETIC-INDUCED CHEMICAL TOXICITY

The use of statistical procedures for the evaluation of data obtained on the effects of drugs and other chemicals tends to obscure the recognition of deviations in response of individual contributors to the data. The investigator may observe an occasional animal which deviates markedly from the majority of his animals in response to a chemical. Such deviants may be disregarded and the data may be discarded because of a variety of unscientific reasons, or the data may be included in the final data. The experimental investigator conventionally applies statistical tests to determine whether his data are sufficiently homogeneous so that statistical methods of analysis of the data are applicable. Ordinarily, unless the deviant data are sizable, such statistical tests for homogeneity of the data may not detect the deviants. For example, the crude data that are acquired for the determination of the LD_{50} of a chemical compound almost never form a true, uniform Gaussian curve when plotted as a frequency–response relationship (Fig. 6.2). Rather, a skewed curve is obtained, and by statistical manipulation the curve is subsequently normalized to give the normal Gaussian form.

The occurrence of a few mutant animals within the group under study may be statistically unimportant because of the small number of animals involved in the study. The discovery of the existence of such mutants

Doses tested (arbitrary units)	1	2	3	4	5	6	7	8	
Animals responding (number)	0	2	1	6	15	14	8	4	50
Animals responding (percent)	0	4	2	12	30	28	16	8	100

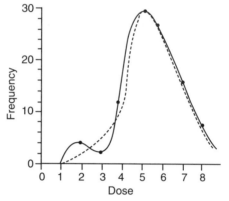

FIGURE 6.2   Graphic representation of data obtained with a hypothetical anesthetic agent in which the dose of the agent required to produce respiratory paralysis was determined in mice. The solid line represents the true curve. The broken line represents the best fitting skewed Gaussian distribution curve.

(abnormal responders) has resulted from recognition that the deviant animals may represent a population separate from the normals. The deviant animals represent mutants and the mutation may be the cause of toxic effects resulting from the administration of agents that are relatively innocuous when given in the same dose to normal members of the population. When such mutants occur and the data are plotted as a frequency–response curve, multiphasic curves are obtained. When such diphasic or triphasic curves are obtained, they are highly suggestive of the existence of mutant animals within the group involved in the study.

Although a mutant that results in the formation of a defective enzyme system may be responsible for the failure of the biologic organism to detoxify a chemical agent, it is entirely possible that the mutant could result in the development of a new, or at least a "more efficient," detoxifying enzyme. In the latter case, if the more efficient enzyme was responsible for detoxication of the chemical agent, then the mutant would protect the organism from the toxicity. If the chemical involved was a drug, then the overall consequence would be not only resistance to any toxic effect of the drug, but also resistance to the therapeutic effect of the drug. However, if the mutant produced a more efficient enzyme and the function of the enzyme was activation (conversion to a more active form) of the agent, then the biologic organism would be liable to exhibit a greater therapeutic, and possibly a greater toxic susceptibility to any given dose of the drug involved. It is also not necessary that the mutant be limited to an enzyme or an enzyme system; rather the mutant can be in the form of an abnormal protein. Such a protein would be one in which the normal amino acid sequence, which identifies the protein, is disrupted by the presence of an incorrect amino acid somewhere along the sequence. If the mutant protein constitutes a target (or receptor) for the foreign chemical, then the protein may exhibit a greater or lower, or even an absence of, affinity for the foreign chemical. Some examples of altered responses to chemical agents due to genetic-based mechanisms are listed in Table 6.1.

For the purpose of categorizing the various toxicologic responses that are the result of mutant enzymes or proteins, it is convenient to identify the toxicity as being (1) the result of a *prolongation* of the action of the agent to the point that it becomes a distinctly detrimental response and there is no accumulation of the agent in the biologic system; (2) the result of repeated exposure to the drug whereby the agent *accumulates* in the biologic system so that concentrations of the agent are reached that will produce toxicity; or (3) the result of a change in the *sensitivity* of the receptor system so that the response represents an altered susceptibility to the chemical agent. This classification of genetic-based toxicity is described more fully below and is followed by some examples.

1. *Prolongation* of the action of a chemical as the result of a deficient biotransformation mechanism, in which case the administered chemical is the primary toxic agent. This condition is exemplified by the prolonged succinylcholine-induced apnea as observed in humans who have a genetically deficient cholinesterase enzyme.

2. *Accumulation* of the chemical as a result of a genetically deficient or absent metabolic transformation mechanism (enzyme system), in which case the administered chemical is the primary toxic agent. This condition would readily occur with drugs that are given in multiple doses at specified intervals. Examples of this condition are the variations between individuals with respect to the acetylation of isoniazid and variations with respect to metabolism of Dicumarol in various members of a given species.

3. *Hypersensitivity,* involving a defective enzyme which causes a borderline level of activity with borderline symptoms of enzyme deficiency when the administered chemical is the primary toxic agent. Examples of this

TABLE 6.1 Altered Responses to Chemicals Due to Genetic-Based Mechanisms

Agent involved [type of drug(s) or chemical(s)]	Mutant involved		Reaction involved [detoxication (D) or activation (A)]	Consequence	Mechanism [prolongation (P), accumulation (A), sensitivity change (S)]
	Type of enzyme or protein	Deficient (D) or more efficient (ME)			
Succinylcholine	Cholinesterase	D	D	Prolonged apnea	P
Succinylcholine	Cholinesterase	ME	D	Drug resistance	
Isoniazid	Acetyl transferase	D	D	Neuropathy	A
Isoniazid	Acetyl transferase	ME	D	Drug resistance	
Hydralazine	Acetyl transferase	D	D	—	
Phenelzine	Acetyl transferase	D	D	—	
Sulfamethazine	Acetyl transferase	D	D	—	
Nitrites	Methemoglobin reduction or abnormal hemoglobin	—	—	Methemoglobinemia	S
Nitrates		—	—	Methemoglobinemia	
Chlorates		—	—	Methemoglobinemia	
Quinones		—	—	Methemoglobinemia	
Methylene blue		—	—	Methemoglobinemia	

Agent	Enzyme / system			Effect	
Primaquine		D	—	Hemolytic anemia	S
Antipyrine	Glucose-6 phosphodehydrogenase, stability of reduced glutathione			Hemolytic anemia	S
Acetanilid (fava beans)		D	—		
Diphenyl hydantoin	Hydroxylation enzyme (vitamin K dependent system?)	D	D	Ataxia, dysarthria	A
Warfarin		ME	—	Drug resistance	
Coumarin	Coumarin hydroxylase (d-amino levulinic acid synthetase)	D	—	Hemorrhage	A
Barbiturates		—	—	Porphyria	
Sulfonamides					
Ethanol	Alcohol dehydrogenase	D	—	Altered metabolism conversion rate	
Ethanol	Alcohol dehydrogenase	ME	—	Drug resistance	
Benzo(a)pyrene	Aryl hydrocarbon hydroxylase	—	A	Resistance to induction of the enzyme	

condition involve the primaquine-induced hemolytic anemia in which there is a genetically altered stability of reduced glutathione and an altered glucose-6-phosphodehydrogenase activity. Additional examples are the abnormal hemoglobins in which there is an altered ability of the hemoglobin to remain in the reduced state, and the sulfonamide and barbiturate-induced porphyrias which are involved with the deficiency of the inhibitor system which normally controls the level of α-amino levulinic acid synthetase.

GENETIC FACTORS IN ACCUMULATION OF CHEMICALS

In the normal human, the antitubercular drug isoniazid undergoes acetylation as one mechanism of metabolic termination of the action of the drug. Formation of the acetylating enzyme is under the influence of a single major gene. Following conventional repeated doses of the compound to a mutant individual who lacks the acetylation gene, the compound can accumulate in the blood. High blood levels of isoniazid are prone to induce the toxicity of polyneuropathy.

Studies of variation between human individuals in regard to metabolism of isoniazid demonstrate the existence of three classes of subjects which may be described as slow, intermediate, and rapid inactivators of the drug. When the blood levels of isoniazid are determined 6 hr after a standard dose of the drug (4 mg/kg) and when these data are plotted as a frequency distribution graph (Fig. 6.3), a trimodal curve is obtained, thereby indicating the three types of subjects. This information, together with observations which indicate that the differences between subjects are not related to

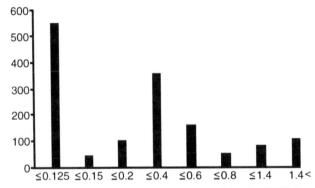

FIGURE 6.3   Frequency distribution curve of 6-hr blood levels of INH (isoniazid) in μg/ml after single dose of 4 mg/kg of INH in 1386 Japanese (from Sunahara, 1961). Data from Motulsky, A. G. (In Steinberg, A. G., and Bearn, A. G., Eds.) *Progress in Medical Genetics,* Grune & Stratton, New York, 1964, p. 52.

differences in intestinal absorption, protein binding, or urinary excretion of the drug, further suggests the existence of a genetically induced deviation from normal. Further investigation disclosed that more of the drug in acetylated form is excreted in the urine in the rapid inactivators. When liver slices of the rapid and slow inactivators were tested for ability to metabolize isoniazid, the compound disappeared at a faster rate in the liver from rapid inactivators. This indicated that the slow inactivators lacked the acetylating enzyme. Genetic studies of families also indicated that the slow inactivators were homozygous. Siblings from slow inactivators always were slow inactivators. Further genetic studies on many populations indicate that the isoniazid-acetylating gene deficiency has the lowest frequency in Eskimos, is common in Negroes and Europeans in general, and is of intermediate frequency in Japanese and Chinese people.

The anticoagulant drug dicumarol undergoes biotransformation in the liver. Failure of such metabolic alteration of the drug would be expected to permit accumulation of the drug following repeated doses, thereby leading to overdose toxicity in the form of hemorrhage. Dicumarol metabolism has been known to vary between members of a species since 1943. The fact that there is also variation in intestinal absorption between animals following oral intake of the drug, together with the demonstration that high doses of the drug would retard the biotransformation rate of the drug initially, cast some doubt on the significance of metabolic variation. Data obtained in subsequent studies of the half-life of the drug in humans still failed to establish that a genetically controlled system was operative in the variation of metabolism of dicumerol. However, studies of families strongly suggest that there are, besides the normal rapid metabolizers, a second group of possible mutants which are slow metabolizers of the drug. Biphasic frequency response curves for dicumarol have been demonstrated.

GENETIC FACTORS IN PROLONGATION OF ACTION OF CHEMICALS

The drug succinylcholine is capable of producing profound, generalized neuromuscular blockade. The intensity of the blockade is dose-dependent, and the action of the drug is terminated by hydrolytic biotransformation induced by the enzyme cholinesterase, which exists in the extracellular fluid of the body. This is a rapid biotransformation process. The average dose of succinylcholine (0.5 to 1 mg/kg) results in a duration of action in the human of not more than 8 to 10 min.

The use of succinylcholine in electroshock therapy to prevent peripheral skeletal muscle convulsive effects disclosed the existence of persons who developed prolonged respiratory paralysis following the administration of doses of the drug. Initial studies of such subjects indicated that they possessed a deficient cholinesterase enzyme system. Subsequent, more intensive investigations have shown that there are persons who are completely lacking in cholinesterase (pseudocholinesterase) enzymes. As a result of many investigations, the conclusion reached is that the prolonged succinylcholine-induced apnea is due to a genetic deficiency in the enzyme involving termination of the action of the drug.

The enzyme pseudocholinesterase is capable of hydrolizing many organic esters and many of these esters are also capable of inhibiting the enzyme by simply increasing the concentration of the ester. When succinylcholine is used as an inhibitor of the enzyme, it can be readily shown that higher concentrations of succinylcholine are required to inhibit the mutant enzyme than are required for inhibition of the normal enzyme. Thus, the enzyme from a mutant subject possesses cholinesterase which is less susceptible to inhibition by succinylcholine, and the mutant enzyme is less capable of hydrolizing succinylcholine. Using the anesthetic dibucaine as the enzyme inhibitor and benzoylcholine as the substrate, the trimodal (normal, deficient, and absent) distribution and the three distinct genotypes of cholinesterase in serum from different persons was demonstrated.

GENETIC FACTORS IN INCREASED SENSITIVITY TO CHEMICALS

Several relatively harmless drugs are known to induce hemolytic anemia in a few members of the population. The antimalarial drug primaquine, an 8-aminoquinoline derivative, is one example of such a drug. Extensive investigations of the primaquine-induced hemolytic anemia have led to the conclusion that this toxicity is due to a genetically controlled red blood cell abnormality which results from an enzyme deficiency. This enzyme deficiency, like the pseudocholinesterase deficiency which is demonstrated only after administering succinylcholine, is a harmless defect unless the system is challenged by certain drugs.

The mechanism of primaquine-induced hemolytic anemia was confusing for 15 years after the introduction of these types of drugs because the drugs also produced methemoglobinemia, a toxicity which was confused with, but not related to, the ultimate mechanism involved with the hemolytic anemia toxicity. The actual demonstration that the defect in the primaquine-sensitive person was localized in the blood cells involved experiments in which the erythrocytes from sensitive individuals were labeled with ^{51}Cr and transfused into nonsensitive recipients who were subsequently given primaquine. Rapid destruction of the primaquine-sensitive cells occurred.

Also, erythrocytes from nonsensitive subjects were given to sensitive subjects who were subsequently given primaquine. The primaquine-sensitive recipients in this latter case hemolyzed their own cells without destroying the transfused (normal) cells. These experiments established that sensitivity to primaquine was not due to abnormal degradation of the drug or to abnormal immune mechanisms in sensitive individuals, and that the defect was in the erythrocyte.

The discovery that reduced glutathione of primaquine-sensitive cells was uniquely sensitive to destruction enabled the development of the "glutathione stability test." This test involved incubation of the red blood cells with acetylphenylhydrazine. This test, when applied to primaquine-sensitive and nonsensitive individuals, readily demonstrated the bimodal distribution of the red-cell-reduced glutathione in the population. Subsequently several groups of investigators established that the sensitive cells also possessed a deficiency in the enzyme glucose-6-phosphate dehydrogenase. It is currently believed that the reduced glutathione instability is the result of a deficiency in glucose-6-phosphate dehydrogenase, although other metabolic lesions may be involved.

The familial and racial nature of the incidence of primaquine sensitivity suggests that the red-cell abnormality is genetically transmitted. Many investigators have shown that the red-cell defect is greater in families of its carriers than in the population at large, that there are less reactor females than males, and that intermediate degrees of deviant glutathione are present in females but not in males. The current concept is that the defect is due to either a sex-linked autosomal gene or a sex-linked gene.

Although several drugs are known to induce hemolytic anemia, the above mechanism has been limited to the primaquine-induced condition. Sulfanilamide- and acetanilid-induced hemolytic anemia appears to be involved with the same mechanism. The chemical, phenylhydrazine, if given in sufficiently high doses, produces hemolytic anemia in all subjects, but primaquine-sensitive subjects are more sensitive to phenylhydrazine. The exact mechanism of action of these drugs on the glucose-6-phosphate dehydrogenase or on the reduced glutathione is not clear, but the evidence indicates that the genetic mutant produces a deficient enzyme which is incapable of maintaining the red blood cell in its normal state when challenged by certain drugs. This system appears to be hypersensitive to the drugs.

DRUG-SENSITIVE HEMOGLOBINS

The drug-sensitive hemoglobins represent additional examples of genetically controlled factors which influence the occurrence of harmful effects from drugs. In the normal animal, the iron in hemoglobin is maintained in the reduced state (as ferrous iron) and remains in the reduced state when combined with oxygen. Oxidation of the iron to the ferric state converts the hemoglobin to methemoglobin. Methemoglobin is not capable of carrying oxygen and therefore fails to carry on one of its main functions, that of oxygen transport in the animal. If sufficient methemoglobin is present (10% in humans), a visible cyanosis is evident. The maintenance of hemoglobin iron in the reduced state in the normal animal is in part accomplished by the presence of the enzyme diaphorase (or methemoglobin reductase).

A variety of chemicals are capable of inducing the formation of methemoglobin, either by a direct stoichiometric action in which 1 mole of the chemical (as exemplified by nitrites) reacts with 1 mole of the hemoglobin to form 1 mole of methemoglobin, or by metabolic transformation to derivatives (as exemplified by conversion of acetanilid to phenylhydroxylamine) which acts directly on the hemoglobin. In the case of phenylhydroxylamine, it reacts with oxyhemoglobin to form nitrosobenzene complexed with hemoglobin and hydrogen peroxide, the latter of which is unstable and yields methemoglobin. The nitrosobenzene is in turn reduced by the enzyme diaphorase, resulting in the reformation of phenylhydroxylamine. Thus, one molecule of phenylhydroxylamine can result in the formation of several molecules of methemoglobin.

The rare clinical condition of hereditary methemoglobinemia has been recognized for over 40 years. The two forms of the disease are: (1) the molecular form in which the molecular structure of hemoglobin differs from the normal hemoglobin, and (2) the enzymatic form in which an enzyme or coenzyme (diaphorase 1) is deficient or absent, and in its absence the normal equilibrium state between hemoglobin and methemoglobin is shifted toward the formation of methemoglobin. Whereas the molecular form of the disease is transmitted as a dominant trait, the enzymatic form is transmitted as a recessive trait by an autosomal recessive gene.

The presence of a genetically deficient mechanism for maintaining the hemoglobin in the reduced state, as exemplified by that condition present in the enzymatic form of hereditary methemoglobinemia, predisposes such mutants to the development of clinical signs of cyanosis when they are administered methemoglobin-forming drugs. Such subjects in the absence of drugs may have from 6 to as much as 50% of their hemoglobin as methemoglobin, and the addition of hemoglobin-oxidizing drugs would be expected to show clinical effects, even though the contribution to the total methemoglobin supplied by the drugs was no greater than that achieved in the normal person. In the case of the mutant exhibiting absence of diaphorase, it is quite unlikely that this mutant would survive doses of acetanilid which would be innocuous in the normal person.

Unlike the enzymatic form of hereditary methemoglobinemia, the mutants exhibiting a molecular deviation involve the type of hemoglobin which does not show increased amounts of methemoglobin in the absence of drugs. The latter mutants are known to be predisposed to severe hemolytic anemia and methemoglobinemia only when challenged by such drugs as the sulfonamides. Two such mutant hemoglobins have been described and have been named after the cities in which the subjects resided (hemoglobin Zurich and hemoglobin Seattle). The alteration of these mutants involves the presence of a histidine residue on the 63rd position of the beta chain on the globin. It is apparent that such mutations in the hemoglobin molecule result in a hemoglobin that is unable to maintain its iron in the reduced state and this condition may lead to methemoglobinemia and possibly hemolytic anemia on administration of oxidizing drugs. Thus, this type of mutant is sensitive to the amounts of drugs which may induce only minor effects on the normal population.

Acute porphyria is an excellent example of a clinical condition that is inherited from a dominant gene according to Mendelian concepts. The condition is characterized by intermittent excretion of porphobilinogen and aminolevulinic acid in the urine and porphyrins in the feces. In humans who have the inherited defect, drugs such as barbiturates and sulfonal will precipitate the condition. Furthermore, several chemicals such as hexachlorobenzene, allyl isopropylacetamide, and certain collidines can induce the condition in experimental animals.

Studies on experimentally induced porphyria using one of the collidines have shown that excretion of the porphyrin precursors results primarily from enhancement of the enzyme activity of aminolevulinic acid (ALA) synthetase in the mitochondria of liver. Normally the liver cells control the porphyrin-synthesizing mechanism by controlling the production of the enzyme ALA-synthetase, which is the first enzyme in the porphyrin biosynthetic chain. When a drug, such as collidine, produces porphyria, it is postulated that the drug will activate the gene for ALA-synthetase by combining with, or inactivating, a repressor control. In the Mendelian disease, it is postulated that an operator gene may be defective and the repression of formation of the ALA-synthetase is held in balance. Therefore, the potential porphyria individual will be highly sensitive to small doses of specific drugs that affect the repressor control system.

GENETIC FACTORS IN SPECIES AND STRAIN RESISTANCE TO TOXICITY

The foregoing discussion pertains to some genetic deviations within a species which may account for increased toxicity from specific drugs or chemicals in relatively few members of the entire population. Genetically induced alterations in metabolic processes in the organism may result in protection of the organism from a harmful effect of a chemical. Such genetic deviations in the levels of "atropinase" in rabbits result in marked protection of the "high atropinase level" animals from the biologic effects of atropine.

Certain members of a species of bacteria may show marked resistance to the biologic effects of specific antibacterial agents which are bacteriocidal or bacteriostatic to the normal majority of that species of bacteria. A similar condition exists in the common house fly, which may be resistant to the lethal effect of the chlorinated hydrocarbon insecticides. Such resistant members of a species probably represent mutants. In either case, it is not well established whether the mutant resistant members of the species existed prior to widespread use of the chemicals, or whether exposure to the chemicals resulted in the development of the mutation, although the latter is strongly suggested in some examples. It is apparent that the resistant mutants could become the comon form of the organism solely because of effective eradication of the susceptible organisms by widespread use of antibacterial or insecticidal chemicals. The occurrence of mutant resistant forms of bacteria and insects is a continuing economic problem, which limits effective control of these organisms by the use of existing antibacterial and insecticidal chemicals. These conditions are considered in greater detail in Chapter 10, The Basis of Selective Toxicity.

It is very probable that there are many as yet undiscovered genetically induced deviants which would account for the rather rare individual who responds untowardly to chemical agents. By systematic investigation of the relatively rare intoxications occurring on the basis of hereditary disposition we may gradually learn of the mechanisms responsible for some of the factors that predispose to chemical intoxication.

CHAPTER 7

Classification of Harmful Effects of Chemicals

The large number of harmful effects that can result from chemical–biological reactions have been classified in the literature by systems (organs), by chemical groups, by types of chemical responses, and by direct and indirect effects of chemicals. Such classifications are frequently designed to consider undesirable effects associated with drug therapy. Drugs represent special types of biologically reactive chemicals which have been studied extensively under both laboratory and clinical conditions. They are intentionally administered, usually in specific doses to humans or at least animals, for the purpose of producing some desired (therapeutic) effect. The desired effect may be the normalizing of an abnormal physiological function, relief of a symptom, eradication of an infection, or destruction of a tumor. In order to achieve this purpose, a drug may produce at the same time undesirable (toxic) effects.

DRUG-INDUCED TOXICITY

Drug toxicities in humans manifest themselves as functional, biochemical, and/or structural changes. Many times the same receptor systems are involved in both the therapeutic and toxic responses. Functional toxicities are due to the pharmacologic effects that are not necessary for the achievement of the desired action of a drug. These funtional toxicities usually occur following conventional doses of the drug and are reversible on discontinuance of the drug. If such changes were not reversible the agent involved would have very restricted use as a drug. Examples of mild forms of these toxicities are the sedation that accompanies antihistamine drug therapy and the psychostimulation that accompanies such drugs as iproniazid. Whereas these changes are mild, functional effects and are reversible on discontinuance of the drug, others may be serious and necessitate withdrawal of the drug from the patient. Examples are the delusions or hallucinations associated with sedative drug use, the cardiac irregularities associated with quinidine therapy, asthma associated with beta adrenergic blocking agents, and edema associated with calcium blocking drugs.

Although all xenobiotic toxicities could be said to be due to fundamental biochemical changes, the functional classification given here defines biochemical toxicity as effects of the drug that do not produce gross or histologic evidence of damage; however, functional symptoms are usually associated with the biochemical damage. Examples are the shifts in hormonal balance accompanying anti-inflammatory hormonal therapy or the shift in acid–base balance associated with aspirin intoxication. Such changes are readily reversible on discontinuance of the drug, provided the normal homeostatic mechanisms are operative in the subjects.

Structural toxicities usually are produced indirectly by biochemical drug effects, but may be classified as toxicities that produce changes in the structure of an organ, tissue, or cell group. Again, such changes may be mild and reversible on discontinuance of the drug. An example is the fatty infiltration of the liver cells associated with chloroform anesthesia or consumption of alcohol. Such structural changes may also be very severe, such as depletion of white blood cells and the sloughing off of the lining of the intestine associated with anticancer drugs. Another good example is phenothiazine-induced cataracts.

All of the foregoing toxicities represent pharmacologic effects that are undesirable, but are known to result from therapeutic doses of the drugs involved. Some appear early in the course of drug therapy, whereas others appear only after continued use of the drug for weeks or months. Therefore, they are toxicities that are *side effects* in reference to the intended effect of the drug. Although side effects of drugs may be said to be dose-related and avoidable by decreasing the dosage of the drug, a decrease in dosage also may result in an unsatisfactory therapeutic effect.

CHEMICALS INTENTIONALLY ADMINISTERED TO BIOLOGIC SPECIMENS

It has been pointed out that drugs belong to the group of *chemicals that are intentionally administered in specific amounts to biologic specimens.* There are many nondrug chemicals that are also intentionally administered to biologic specimens in specific amounts, some of which are not necessarily intended for administration to all species. The most obvious of such chemicals would be nutrient substances which consist of complex organic food substances such as the proteins, carbohydrates, and fats, and the accessory food substances such as inorganic salts and vitamins. The respiratory gases would also be included in this category. Less obvious members of this category are food additives (preservatives), drugs, and cosmetics, as well as pesticides and insecticides, exposure to which may be limited to certain species of biologic specimens. In the case of drugs, the dose is regulated to minimize undesirable effects from the drug, and in the case of insecticides the dose is regulated to be excessive only to the uneconomic species.

CHEMICALS NOT INTENDED FOR ADMINISTRATION TO BIOLOGIC SPECIMENS

Chemicals that are intentionally administered to biologic specimens cannot be compared with a second category comprising *chemicals that are not intended for introduction into biologic specimens,* basically because there is no dose or concentration for use of the latter group in order to achieve a specific purpose. Thousands of chemicals are available in the form of pure agents or mixtures of agents and range from household products to industrial–occupational chemicals, or nonfood botanical specimens. The majority of these substances fundamentally are not intended for introduction into biologic systems. Exposure to these agents is frequently unavoidable, and when such compounds do gain access to biologic specimens through incidental, accidental, or intentional exposure, any dose of the chemical capable of producing an untoward effect would be considered an overdose.

EXPECTED OR NORMAL EFFECTS OF CHEMICALS

With drugs as well as with all other chemicals, effects that can be repeatedly induced in biologic specimens become known as expected effects whether they are therapeutic or toxic; they might also be considered the *normal effects* of the chemical. The incidence of occurrence of these effects is primarily dose-dependent, although the dose required to achieve these effects may be different between species or within members of a species. These normal effects do not require any form of preconditioning exposure to the chemical. Thus, if the dose is great enough, the effect occurs in virtually all animals exposed to the chemical. It should be recognized that a large number of factors play a part in the degree of hyper- or hyposensitivity of specific biologic specimens to any given chemical, and some of these factors are considered in other chapters in this book. Normal effects of xenobiotic chemicals on biologic tissue may be said to occur in any biologic specimen which inherently has the target system in the tissue which the foreign chemical is capable of influencing directly or indirectly. To clarify the foregoing statement, one would not expect a xenobiotic agent that reacted only with hemoglobin to produce the same effect on a biologic specimen that had no hemoglobin, but if the two biologic species had identical structures, a foreign chemical which directly affected that type of structure would be expected to produce a similar effect on the two species.

The intensity of effect of all chemicals that are capable of affecting biologic tissues is related directly to the concentration of the chemical that gains access to the target site in the tissue. Therefore, all normal toxic effects of chemicals are the result of overdose or excessive concentrations of the chemical. The toxic concentration necessary for one species may be greatly different from that for a second species, but since there is, for any chemical, a concentration sufficiently low to be harmless to the majority of the population, this concentration is generally considered an acceptable nontoxic concentration. If some members of the population respond excessively to the acceptable dose or concentration of the chemical, then that member is said to be hypersensitive, in a toxicologic sense, to the chemical. Hypersensitivity therefore is manifested as an excessive, normal, expected effect that is induced by a normal dose or concentration of a chemical in some members of a supposedly uniform population of biologic specimens. Therefore in a hypersensitive subject the normal dose, or even less than the normal dose, of a chemical represents an excessive dose.

UNEXPECTED OR ABNORMAL EFFECTS OF CHEMICALS

A basic classification of types of toxicities from chemicals should not be limited to drugs, but rather should be applicable to all chemicals. Such a classification could be based on the fact that toxicity is essentially an unwanted effect that is produced on a biologic specimen by a chemical. All toxic effects can be conveniently divided into two principal types based on whether or not the effect is one that involves preconditioning of the biologic specimen. The effects that involve no preconditioning of the specimen are the *expected* or *normal* effects described above, and the effects that involve preconditioning of the animal may be called the *unexpected* or *abnormal* toxic effects. Abnormal toxic effects are not pharmacologic effects or side effects that can be induced in the majority of members of a population of a species by simply increasing the dose of the chemical. Normal effects of chemicals, as described here, differ from the abnormal effects primarily in that the latter effects involve preconditioning (sensitization) of the biologic specimen to the chemical, in which case an immunologic mechanism is responsible for the toxicity.

The foregoing has indicated that for the purpose of developing a mechanistic classification of harmful effects of all chemicals (Table 7.1) there are four primary considerations that are pertinent: (1) all chemicals can be divided into two categories according to whether or not the chemical is intended for introduction into biologic specimens, (2) all effects of chemicals on biologic specimens can be divided into two categories depending upon whether the response is a normal or abnormal response, (3) all effects of chemicals are dose-dependent, and (4) there are biologic variations between species and within species in response to specific chemicals.

TABLE 7.1 Classification of Mechanisms of Harmful Effects of Chemicals

A. Chemicals *not* intended for introduction into biologic systems
  1. Normal effects depending on:
    a. Nonspecific caustic or corrosive actions
    b. Specific toxicologic actions
    c. Production of pathological sequelae
  2. Abnormal effects depending on:
    a. Immune mechanisms
B. Chemicals intended for introduction into biologic systems
  1. Normal effects associated with:
    a. Exposure to normal doses or concentrations and depending on:
      (1) Malfunction of mechanisms for terminating action of the agent
      (2) Actions on the wrong target system
      (3) Synergism with other chemicals
    b. Exposure to excessive doses or concentrations and depending on:
      (1) Nonspecific caustic or corrosive actions
      (2) Exaggerated pharmacologic effects
      (3) Specific toxicologic actions
      (4) Production of pathological sequelae
      (5) Sociologic complications
  2. Abnormal effects depending on:
    a. Immune mechanisms

It may be noted in Table 7.1 that harmful effects of chemicals that are intended for introduction into biologic systems may be associated with ordinary doses or excessive doses of the chemical. In the case of chemicals not intended for introduction into biologic systems, any dose that was capable of producing a harmful effect would be considered an excessive dose. Division of all chemicals into these two classes is proper only from the viewpoint of the toxicologist who is interested in harmful chemical–biologic reactions and interactions. The division of all chemicals into these two groups is not satisfactory to the chemist, neither is it a satisfactory division for the pharmacologist or biologist. The commonly encountered category of idiosyncratic reactions (reactions dependent on an individual example and for which no known mechanism is recognized) purposely has been omitted with the belief that as mechanisms of action become understood for any compound, they will fit into one or another of the categories listed in the classification. The classification presented does not attempt to categorize the "specific toxicologic effects," because such effects are numerous and varied and may be obtained for most compounds from the standard references listed in Chapter 15. Some examples of specific toxicologic effects constitute entire volumes. The following two chapters consist of a discussion of the normal and abnormal effects of chemicals and some examples of each type of effect.

CHAPTER 8

Normal Toxic Effects of Chemicals

HARMFUL EFFECTS OF CHEMICALS NOT INTENDED FOR INTRODUCTION INTO BIOLOGIC SYSTEMS

Although there are many chemicals that are not intended for introduction into biologic systems, most such chemicals have been produced for use by humans. Proper labeling of solids, liquids, and gases and control of transportation of those agents that have a high order of potential toxicity are required by federal regulatory agencies so that ready recognition and due respect will be accorded these agents. The presence of foreign chemicals in contaminated atmospheric environments as well as in food substances and in potable water makes many such chemicals available to biologic tissue. Undue exposure of humans to such chemicals is usually incidental or accidental in nature, but may be intentional when such agents are used with suicidal intent, or for recreation.

Nonspecific Caustic or Corrosive Actions

When toxicity in humans occurs on contact with xenobiotic chemicals, the toxicity may be manifested at the site of exposure, that is, on the skin or in the respiratory tract. Frequently, such toxicity is the result of the caustic or corrosive nature of the chemical. Such agents are commonly referred to as "primary irritants" because they induce local, minor to severe inflammatory response or even extensive necrosis of the tissue cells in direct relation to the concentration available to the tissue. This action is nonspecific and occurs on all cells regardless of type. Strong inorganic or organic acids or bases are the most common examples of a substance which by definition is capable of producing a chemical "burn" at the site of contact. However, such effects may be induced by compounds that are not necessarily strong acids or bases. For example, the refrigerant methylbromide is an excellent methylating agent for organic synthesis; if applied to the skin or mucous membranes or inhaled in the respiratory system it will produce chemical burns of an intensity directly related to the exposure concentration. Gases such as sulfur dioxide and nitrogen dioxide, which are converted respectively to sulfurous and nitrous acid in the presence of water (at membranes or in the air), produce a primary irritant effect. Such agents may be encountered in smog (smoke–fog) conditions in urban areas where coal and fuel oil are used extensively. The aldehydes, such as acrolein (allyl aldehyde) and formaldehyde, are strong irritants to mucous membranes.

The primary irritants that are inhaled into the respiratory tract of animals have no greater action in the lungs than on the skin, but less severe effects on the alveolar tissue may lead to serious consequences because of edema in the lungs with loss of air space and impaired transfer of respiratory gases. In an animal with lung disease and only a borderline reserve of functional capacity, exposure to primary irritants in amounts that may be tolerated in the normal animal may lead to serious impairment of function.

Specific Toxicologic Actions

In contrast to the nonspecific action of the primary irritants, other compounds may have a high degree of specificity, so that they will react at low dose levels only at certain receptor sites. One of the most potent agents known belongs to this group of substances. It is botulinus toxin, a high-molecular-weight globulin-like protein produced in the several groups of *Clostridium botulinum* bacteria. On the basis of lethal effect in the rat, the estimated lethal dose of botulinus toxin for an average adult human is approximately 0.01 μg. Botulinus toxin owes its toxicity to an action at certain nerve terminals whereby it prevents liberation of the neurohumor responsible for nerve to muscle transfer of impulses. Symptomatology is primarily that of paralysis of muscle function. The specific toxicologic effects of compounds in this group of chemicals may be either reversible or irreversible in nature, depending primarily on the dose. The effect of botulinus toxin is reversible in time if the animal has enough muscle function remaining to enable it to maintain its respiratory metabolic requirements throughout the symptom phase of the toxicity.

Chemicals in this group may have a high degree of specificity of action, which causes an initial effect on function of the organism and a subsequent pathological change in specific organs. Examples are the hepatotoxicity from the chlorinated hydrocarbons, such as carbon tetrachloride and dichlormethane, or the optic nerve damage that occurs in primates and is associated with methyl alcohol or a metabolite of methyl alcohol. In the above examples, exposure to greater concentrations of each agent would be expected to produce excessive organ damage. If the effect involves organic damage to tissue, then sequelae consistent with the degree of tissue damage would be expected to follow exposure to the chemical. The degree of permanent pathologic sequelae which would occur following intoxication with this group of chemicals is dependent on the efficiency of the repair mechanisms involved and on the type of tissue under consideration.

Certain tissues that have been structurally and functionally damaged by a toxic chemical may undergo healing by the process of regeneration whereby the dead cells are replaced with new cells, or if the cells were not sufficiently damaged, structure and function may return to normal in the same cells. In contrast to this, the damaged cells may be replaced with fibrous tissue (scar tissue), in which case the pathological sequelae involve the formation of a permanently altered tissue.

In contrast to chemicals that have nonspecific irritant actions and chemicals that have specific actions at receptor sites, certain additional agents are essentially biologically inactive. Examples of such agents are the inert gases and vapors such as neon, nitrous oxide, helium, methane and ethane. When such agents are present in sufficiently high concentrations in air to displace oxygen, the oxygen-dependent animals become hypoxic in direct proportion to the degree of oxygen deficit. Such gases are therefore properly termed asphyxiants. Unintentional, acute exposure of humans to high concentrations of these agents occurs without warning, since these agents are odorless and nonirritant. Toxicity from such agents is therefore indirectly induced, and acute as well as chronic pathological effects consequent to oxygen deprivation are again the result of a dose–response relationship.

Specific toxicologic effects that are irreversible, particularly when they are life threatening, include teratogenesis, mutagenesis, and carcinogenesis. Exposure to xenobiotics that produce any of these effects as an ordinary consequence of their actions must be limited. However, many compounds do not clearly fall in or out of these categories, particularly when the question concerns clinical toxicology. In general, in the absence of strongly positive clinical experience with any compound, toxicologists rely on a battery of laboratory animal and *in vitro* tests to demonstrate whether any compound may or may not produce these toxicities. From these data an estimate is made regarding the risk involved when humans are exposed to the compound.

Although there is no generally recognized and accepted list of compounds that are known mutagens in humans, compounds that are carcinogenic via a direct action on the genetic mechanism could be classified as mutagens. That is, many carcinogenic compounds are also mutagens and there are recognized lists of carcinogenic compounds. The United States Department of Health and Human Services, through the National Toxicology Program, publishes annually a listing of carcinogenic substances. The 1994 report summary lists two categories of substances or groups of substances. One category consists of 24 substances for which evidence from human studies indicates that there is a causal relationship between exposure and human cancer. The second category consists of 156 substances which may reasonably be anticipated to be carcinogens, defined as those substances for which there is limited evidence of carcinogenicity in humans or sufficient evidence of carcinogenicity in experimental animals. Table 8.1 consists of selected substances from the above categories

TABLE 8.1 A Selected List of Carcinogenic Substances (A) in Humans and (B) in Animals

A	B
Aflatoxins	Acetaldehyde
Asbestos	2-Acetylaminofluorene
Arsenic	Butylated hydroxyanisole
Benzene	Carbon tetrachloride
Benzidine	Chloroform
Chromium	Dimethylsulfate
Conjugated estrogens	Estrogens (not conjugated)
Mustard gas	Formaldehyde
2-Napthylamine	Lead acetate
Vinyl chloride	Phenacetin
	Polyaromatic hydrocarbons (PAHs)
	Saccharin
	Safrole
	Thiourea
	Urethane

Note. From Seventh Annual Report on Carcinogens, 1994, Summary, U.S. Dept. Health and Human Services, National Toxicology Program, P.H.S. See text for definitions of A and B.

showing the diverse and unrelated nature of compounds that produce cancer.

A teratogen can be properly defined as a chemical that increases the occurrence of structural or functional abnormalities in offspring if administered to either parent before conception, to the female during pregnancy, or directly to the developing organism. The time of exposure of the fetus generally determines the nature of the teratogenic defect. A teratogen may be active in one species but not in another. For example, cortisone is commonly used to study cleft palate in experimental animals but it is not considered teratogenic in humans. Also, a biotransformation product of a xenobiotic agent may be responsible for a teratogenic action. A good example of this is the drug thalidomide, for which there is some evidence that a metabolic product of thalidomide is the responsible teratogen. It is also recognized that a teratogenic effect may be induced indirectly by a xenobiotic agent by creating a metabolic disturbance in the female during gestation. Ethyl alcohol is a possible example of this type of teratogenic agent. Table 8.2 is a selected list of agents known to be teratogenic in humans and the main teratogenic effects that are produced by each agent.

The Concept of Pathologic Sequelae

Pathologic sequelae are those permanent malfunctions or malformations of tissue that remain after exposure to the chemical agent has been discontinued but which were initially caused by the chemical. An excellent example of a pathologic sequel is scar tissue, which is fibrous tissue that results from failure of normal cells to regenerate following laceration or burning of the skin. Severe chemical burns can result in the production of such scar

TABLE 8.2   A Selected List of Teratogenic Agents in Humans and Their Principle Effects

Compound	Clinical effects
Thalidomide	Limb anomalies
Ethyl alcohol	Growth retardation, cranio-facial defects
Diethylstilbestrol	Clear cell carcinoma in young adult females
Cocaine	Limb and urinary tract defects, congenital heart disease
Organic mercury	Fetal "Minamata disease," cerebral palsy
Trimethadone	Cleft palate, cardiac anomalies
Aminopterin	Hydrocephalis, facial deformities

Note. Modified from Shepard, T.H., *Catalog of Teratogenic Agents,* 7th ed., Johns Hopkins Press, 1992.

tissue. Chemically induced cancer is also a good example of a pathologic sequel that can become evident long after exposure to certain chemical carcinogens has occurred. However, more subtle forms of pathologic sequelae can occur following exposure to certain chemicals. For example, inhalation of excessive amounts of tricresyl phosphate or methyl butyl ketone as well as hexane has been reported to lead to the destruction of certain nerve cells, so that after exposure to the agents has been discontinued, residual muscle paralysis remains. In humans, ingestion of methylmercury as a contaminant of food is known to produce mental retardation which persists after the chemical is no longer in the body. In a similar manner, undue exposure of humans to the herbicide paraquat can lead to a change in lung tissue that continues to develop long after exposure to the agent has been discontinued. In each of the foregoing examples, it is almost certain that the initial effect of the chemical on the biologic tissue occurred at the time of exposure to the chemical and the subsequent pathologic sequel that developed was the result of failure of the tissue to regenerate normal cells. Such initial changes are biochemical in nature and they go undetected until the easily measurable structural changes become manifest, at which time the term "pathologic sequelae" is applicable.

HARMFUL EFFECTS OF CHEMICALS INTENDED FOR INTRODUCTION INTO BIOLOGIC SYSTEMS

Toxicity Associated with Normal Concentrations

Whenever a chemical is developed in the laboratory or extracted from a natural source and placed in the environment so that it becomes identified, some form of biologic specimen should be expected to come in contact with the chemical. However, many chemicals are developed expressly for use on biologic tissue, either for their desirable effects or for their harmful effects. Drugs are developed for the beneficial effects that may be achieved by their proper use. Pesticides and insecticides are presumed to be developed for the indirect beneficial effects on an economic species by virtue of their harmful effect on one or more uneconomic species. Ironically, some chemicals are even developed for war purposes with the objective of achieving either an incapacitating or lethal effect on an enemy. Cosmetics and food additives, such as antibacterial substances, antioxidants, flavors, and sweetening agents, are only a few of the many chemicals that are intended to be introduced into biologic systems.

Drugs are good examples of chemicals that are intended for use by humans. A characteristic of all drugs is that there is some established amount (or dose) as well as schedule of amounts (if the drug is one that is to be taken on repeated occasions) that represents an acceptable and recognized quantity that can be used with confidence that harmful effects will at least not occur frequently. However, even ordinary doses of drugs produce undesirable "side actions." The frequency of occurrence of such side actions is listed in the package inserts that come with the drug. Such side actions may become intolerable and even lethal.

All chemicals have specific limits in regard to the amount that can be used without producing undesired effects. These limits obviously must include wide margins of safety as far as the economic species is concerned. Even when the intended use of the chemical is to induce a toxic effect or death in an uneconomic species, precautions are observed by the user. Thus the toxicity of all chemicals in this group becomes important regardless of their intended use, especially when the economic species is the human. In earlier chapters, it has been pointed out that various biologic as well as chemical factors influence the biologic effect of all chemicals, and that variations in response to specific amounts of chemicals are ever prevalent in the biologic kingdom. Most conditions that give rise to toxic effects from amounts (or doses) of chemicals that are tolerated by the majority of a population can be ascribed to known mechanisms, or if enough information is available regarding such reactions, they would be expected to fit in one of the categories listed in Table 7.1.

It has already been mentioned that idiosyncratic toxic reactions to chemicals, that is, reactions supposedly due to unknown factors inherent in individuals, most certainly occur, but this terminology is purposely avoided here; as additional information becomes available such reactions seem to fit in the categories listed in Table 7.1.

Many of the toxic reactions that occur with this group of chemicals following normal doses involve drugs or pesticides, and the mechanisms have become clarified as a result of studies which were performed because of the occurrence and importance of the toxicities in humans.

Toxicity Due to Malfunction of Mechanisms for Terminating Action of the Agent. The most obvious cause of toxicity from normal doses of a chemical is a malfunction of the mechanism responsible for terminating the action of the agent. Under this condition, normal doses would be present for a longer period of time in the animal, and repeated doses would be likely to result in accumulation of the chemical to toxic levels in the animal. An example of such an effect would be the accumulation, as a result of kidney disease, of drugs that are ordinarily terminated by excretion in the urine. The antibiotic drug tetracycline, following conventional repeated dosage, rapidly accumulates in the human when kidney function is seriously impaired, and this accumulation has been known to cause death. Impairment of a biotransformation mechanism involved in detoxication of a chemical also would interfere with termination of action of the chemical. This may result from a genetic deviation in the subject (see Chapter 6) or from the presence of other chemicals that may inhibit the detoxication enzyme mechanism (see Chapter 4).

The presence of other drugs may influence the termination of action of a specific agent and thereby influence toxicity of the specific agent. An example is that of feeding tyramine (in cheese) to an animal that has been pretreated with a monoamine oxidase inhibitor. In this case the monoamine oxidase inhibitor inhibits the enzyme (monoamine oxidase) which is normally present in the intestinal wall and normally inactivates tyramine as it is being absorbed from the food in the gastrointestinal tract. The result is accumulation of tyramine in the circulation in sufficient amounts to produce undesirable cardiovascular effects. However, that tyramine is the sole agent responsible for the toxicity in such cases has not been fully established.

The adsorption of a drug on plasma proteins is basically a mechanism of inactivation or temporary removal of the drug from its active state in the animal. Displacement of one drug by another from protein carrier sites can lead to rapid increases in the free form of the first drug, thereby inducing toxicity from the first drug. A good example of this is the fact that the anticoagulant drug warfarin can be displaced from nonspecific binding sites on plasma proteins by phenylbutazone, to the extent that spontaneous hemorrhage may occur. Also, the anti-folic acid agent methotrexate is displaced by sulfonamides and salicylates, and since methotrexate is generally employed in amounts that approach seriously toxic tissue levels, such displacement could lead to toxicity due to methotrexate.

A malfunction of biotransformation mechanisms for terminating the action of several drugs exists in infants. Infants not only are immature in age, but are generally biochemically immature. Certain newborn rabbits, mice, and guinea pigs lack the microsomal systems that are present in the adult animals. Both the duration of sedative action and the lethal toxicity of hexobarbital have been shown to decrease with age in the animal, and to correlate well with the level of microsomal enzyme activity for detoxifying the drug. In contrast to the infant, the aged and debilitated subject presents a biologic specimen that is metabolically deficient. In these patients, a chemical that pharmacologically impairs physical or mental activity begins its action on an already imperfect system, so that small amounts of drug effect may be excessive.

Toxicity Due to Action on the Wrong Target System. Harmful effects of a drug may result from an effect of the drug on the wrong target organ or receptor system. All drugs are imperfect, and no drug is so selective in its action that it will have but one action on the biologic specimen. The oncolytic drugs and antibiotic drugs are good examples of this type of toxicity. The inhibitory effects of the oncolytic drugs on rapidly proliferating cells is the reason for their usefulness in the treatment of malignancies, but at present these agents are not sufficiently selective in action because they also inhibit rapidly proliferating cells that are desirable, such as cells in the intestinal mucosa, in the bone marrow, and in the testis. The effect of the oncolytic agents on these desirable cells is essentially an effect of the drug on the wrong target organ.

The high order of therapeutic efficiency of some of the antibiotic drugs when they are used in the treatment of bacterial infections not only leads to death of the invading bacteria but also leads to death of some desirable bacteria in the host, thereby promoting the development of superinfections. Such superinfections are infections caused by the growth of resistant organisms (bacteria, lichens, or fungi) that are normally held in check by the forms of bacteria normally present in the oral and intestinal tracts of the host animals. Therefore, superinfections that occur during antibiotic therapy result from effects of the antibiotic on the wrong target system.

Most side actions of drugs are essentially actions of the drugs on the wrong target organ. Usually, the side actions of a drug determine the allowable dose. If it were not for the side actions of morphine on the gut and the respiratory center of the brain, the normal doses of morphine could be increased indefinitely.

All drugs have side effects, and the occurrence of exaggerated side effects either directly or indirectly as a result of the use of a drug indicates toxicities of the drug. Skin and corneal pigmentation, development of Parkinson's tremors, and hepatic dysfunction with jaundice resulting from the use of chlorpromazine are side effects that can become excessive and necessitate discontinuance of the drug. Suppression of thyrotropic hormone is a side effect associated with adrenocorticoid therapy and can become serious and require discontinuance of the drug. Teratogenic actions of drugs are side effects that are actions of drugs on the wrong target organ, namely the fetus. Thus, thalidomide is a good sedative drug, even in the pregnant woman, but if it is administered to the pregnant woman at the improper interval after conception, it is likely to induce malformations in the developing fetus.

Toxicity Due to Synergism with Other Chemicals. Harmful effects of a chemical associated with normal dosage of the chemical can occur as a result of the presence of other drugs that have similar pharmacologic actions. The total effect of two agents that have similar pharmacologic actions is a response that is either equal to the summation of the effects of the individual agents or greater than the summation of the independent effects of the two agents. The former condition is aptly termed "summation." The latter response is termed "potentiation" or "synergism" and represents the condition whereby one drug is made more potent in the presence of an amount of another drug which alone may produce minimal or no pharmacologic effect. The classic example of this is the potentiation of epinephrine response in the laboratory animal by the addition of cocaine.

Usually, the effect of two agents is the summation of the responses to each agent. An example of summation of action of two drugs is the enhancement of sedation as produced by an antihistaminic agent when barbiturates are administered. Summation of drug action is commonly encountered in regard to the use of anesthetic agents. Preanesthetic medication may consist of a sedative (such as a barbiturate), and when this is followed with general inhalation anesthesia (such as nitrous oxide, ether, or cyclopropane) the total dose of the inhaled anesthetic is less than that required in the absence of the preanesthetic medication. In these cases, the threshold required to produce a given intensity of pharmacologic effect by a second drug is lowered because of the presence of the initial drug. Attention has been directed toward the summation or potentiation that takes place among the various pesticides in regard to lethal response of mixtures of these agents. The hypokalemia that is associated with the clinical use of organomercurial diuretic agents may enhance the cardiac toxicity of the digitalis glycosides. Physiological imbalance in acid–base status, as well as dehydration of animals created by excessive vomiting or diarrhea that may be drug induced, increases the toxicity of improper ion therapy.

The list of direct and indirect effects that one chemical can have on the toxicity of a second chemical is almost limitless. Chemical-induced disease resulting in impairment of function of an organ can markedly influence the toxicity of a subsequently administered agent that has a similar action, and can influence the termination of action of a second agent that may have a completely different pharmacologic action. For example, in industry permanent injury to the respiratory airway, such as the pulmonary fibrosis and emphysema associated with chronic exposure to dusts or primary irritants, or damage to the liver and kidney associated with exposure to the chlorinated hydrocarbons, impairs the reserve capacity of the organ to carry on its function; if the organ is then exposed to additional agents that have a primary toxic effect on the same organ, small degrees of toxicities may be sufficient to seriously impair the remaining function of the organ. Mercurial-induced disease in the kidney predisposes the organ to toxicity from subsequent exposures to arsenic. Industrial workers with various degrees of exposure to benzene may show a direct toxicity in hematopoietic tissue, manifested as diminution in erythrocytes; some subjects even show a reduction in hemoglobin. These subjects would be expected to be susceptible to methemoglobin-forming agents, such as nitrites, or oxygen-displacing agents, such as carbon monoxide.

Toxicity Associated with Excessive Concentrations

Nonspecific Caustic or Corrosive Actions. Exposure to excessive doses or concentrations of chemicals intended for administration to biologic specimens can induce toxic effects of the same type as those described for the chemicals not intended for introduction into biologic systems. Caustic or corrosive chemicals intended for introduction into biologic systems are usually agents used as bacteriocides or fungicides, e.g., cresol; mercurials such as thimerosal (Merthiolate) and merbromin (Mercurochrome); inorganic compounds such as silver nitrate, mercuric chloride, and iodine; the quaternary ammonia compounds such as benzalkonium and cetylpyridinium; and the acids such as boric acid. When these agents are used in proper concentrations on surfaces or skin, they serve a useful purpose as antiseptics or germicides, although it is generally agreed that when these substances are used on the human skin, they are not capable of sterilizing the skin without destroying it. Accidental or intentional consumption of these agents by animals can cause local effects ranging from primary irritation to gross necrosis of the tissue in the gastrointestinal tract as well as systemic effects.

Exaggerated Pharmacologic or Toxicologic Actions. Excessive doses of drugs that affect physiological mechanisms can produce toxicity either by excessive pharmacologic effect or by specific toxic actions or side actions, which are ordinarily avoided by proper, intelligent use of drugs. An example of the former is the excessive and possibly lethal pharmacologic effect that occurs when barbiturates or tranquilizers are taken for suicidal purposes. Examples of the latter are the excessive toxicity produced by the cardiac glycosides on cardiac function and the hemorrhagic episodes associated with the use of anticoagulant drugs when therapy with these drugs is not properly conducted or followed. An additional important type of excessive exposure involves accidental or intentional exposure of the wrong target species, that is, the economic species, to agents such as the commonly available potent pesticides and insecticides which are used for their high order of toxicity to the uneconomic species.

Pathologic Sequelae.   In order for a chemical compound to be included in the group of chemicals intended for introduction into biologic systems, it should not produce serious pathologic sequelae at least in an economic species, except possibly under unwarranted conditions of abusive use of the chemical. However, there have been several instances in which serious pathologic sequelae occurred after chemical agents were already in use even by humans. In some of these cases, acceptable as well as excessive doses initiated the pathology. An example is the carcinogenic agent butter yellow, which had been used as a food coloring agent. Another example is the sedative drug thalidomide, which was found to be a potent teratogenic agent when administered at the proper time to pregnant women. Also, the drug triparanol was found to produce cataracts in man after it had been in use for several years. Such sequelae obviously result from the action of the chemical on the wrong target system; they are composed of toxicities that are essentially irreversible. Whenever serious pathologic sequelae such as teratogenic, mutagenic, or carcinogenic effects are discovered in an economic species, restrictions are placed on the use of the agent. Whenever a new chemical agent is intended for use as a food additive or a drug, it should be thoroughly tested through the use of preclinical toxicity tests for its ability to produce pathologic sequelae.

Sociologic Factors in Toxicity.   Certain drugs, such as those that influence the functions of the brain, acquire considerable importance more for sociologic reasons than for their therapeutic value. Notable among these are the narcotics, barbiturates, amphetamines, and alcohol. Their sociologic significance stems from the fact that certain people become addicted to their use, and society (in the United States) disapproves of addiction to such drugs. Pharmacologically, addiction evolves through the following conditions: first, habituation, which is the psychologic or emotional dependency on the drug; second, physical dependence, whereby an altered physiological state exists because of frequent exposure to the drug and withdrawal of the drug leads to a physical and emotional illness known as the abstinence or withdrawal syndrome; and third, tolerance to many of the pharmacologic effects of the drug.

It is unlikely that without tolerance, which leads to the use of greater than normal doses of the drug, a person could ever become addicted to these agents. This is because ordinary doses would fail to produce a desired pharmacologic effect, which is important in maintaining the compulsion to take the drug. It is for this reason that the toxic effect (in a sociologic sense) of addiction to drugs is placed in the category of harmful effects of excessive dosage of chemicals intended for exposure to biologic specimens. It may be argued that addiction should not be considered as a harmful effect of such drugs because the addict who is able to obtain the drug may carry on normal activities and be physically normal. If direct organic or functional toxicity occurs in addicts, it may be said to occur only under conditions in which the chemical is withdrawn from the subject, thereby leading to the abstinence syndrome.

The *abnormal* effects of those chemicals that are intended for introduction into biologic systems are also associated with the development in the biologic system of immune mechanisms. These mechanisms, together with examples, are discussed in Chapter 9.

Abnormal Response to Chemicals

Physicians frequently use the terms "hypersensitivity reactions" and "sensitization reactions" interchangeably to describe chemical-induced effects that are attributable to the immune mechanism in the body. It would be preferable to reserve the term "hypersensitivity" to describe a response with the following characteristics: (1) it occurs in only a few individuals, (2) it consists of the normal, expected effects of the chemical, (3) it does not require preconditioning of the individual to the chemical, and (4) it occurs following the administration of a dose of a compound that is smaller than the usual dose. That is, a hypersensitive response also may be defined as a normal pharmacologic or toxicologic response of greater intensity than that which occurs in the majority of the population following a given dose of the chemical agent.

In contrast to this, a sensitization reaction to a chemical is the response involving the immune mechanism. It is an abnormal effect of the chemical in the sense that it is different from the pharmacologic effect associated with ordinary doses or the toxicologic effect resulting from excessive doses of the chemical.

THE IMMUNE MECHANISM

The immune mechanism is a natural defense system present in mammals. It is a defense system in the sense that it protects the body from invading microbes and chemicals that have antigenic properties. An antigen by definition is any substance that activates the immune system leading to the production of proteins called antibodies. Antibodies can be unattached to cells or can be attached to cell membranes. Once formed by the initial exposure to the antigen the antibodies recognize any subsequent exposures to the antigen. A resultant antigen–antibody interaction takes place. If the antigen is a microbe (or part of one) the immune system destroys the microbe or facilitates destruction of the microbe via other cells (phagocytes) that the reaction recruits. Actually, one antibody can unite with different antigens and one antigen with many antibodies, in both cases with varying degrees of affinity. In such a manner the body develops "immunity," such as immunity to small pox by exposure to a small pox-like virus (cow pox virus).

A very important property of the normal immune system is that it is capable of recognizing "foreign" chemicals (such as xenobiotic agents) as being different from "self" chemicals. When the system fails in this regard self chemicals may initiate the immune mechanism. When this happens the subjects develop autoimmune disease, that is, immunity against their own cells. The immune system is therefore a two-step process, the first being formation of antibody associated with the initial exposure and the second being the antigen–antibody interaction associated with subsequent exposure to the antigen. Many xenobiotic chemicals are probably incomplete antigens (called haptenes) and bind to macromolecules in the body in order to become antigens.

The immune mechanism involves the following events: the initial exposure to a chemical substance, an induction period in the animal, and finally the production of a new protein called an antibody (Fig. 9.1). As illustrated in Fig. 9.1, the chemical or a metabolic product of the chemical acts as a *haptene* (or hapten), a substance that combines with an endogenous protein to form an *antigen*. An antigen is capable of eliciting the formation of cellular or humoral new proteins called *antibodies*. The initial exposures do not result in cellular damage but cause the animal to be "sensitized" to subsequent exposures to the chemical. Exposure of the animal to the chemical on a subsequent occasion will lead to the formation of the antigen, which reacts with the preformed antibodies leading to a cellular response or even cellular damage. This is the "immune response" or "allergic response."

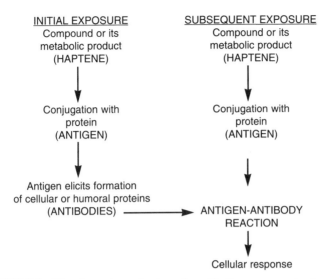

FIGURE 9.1 The allergenic mechanism of sensitization responses to chemicals.

INITIAL EXPOSURE TO HAPTENS—THE
SENSITIZING SYSTEMS

The basic components of the immune system have been described in detail. A brief description of the system is helpful to understand the classification of what the "abnormal effects of chemicals" are and how they are produced by xenobiotic chemicals. Initially it is clear that not all but many chemicals are potential antigens. Those that are antigens (or fragments of which are antigens) when allowed to enter the body encounter specific cells (lymphocytes) in the blood that recognize any conceivable antigen. This process is aided by additional "accessory" cells which physically take the chemical antigen to sites in the body, mainly the spleen and lymph nodes, where there is an abundance of lymphocytes and where those lymphocytes are "activated" by recognizing the antigen. Activation causes the cell to produce antibodies and to collaborate with other nonantigen producing cells (i.e., phagocytes) and with proteins (termed "compliments") in an all-out attempt to inactivate the antigen. The immune system is under continuous self-regulation, enabling it to regulate the intensity of the immune response to the antigenic load that it encounters.

The activation of a lymphocyte leading to the production of an immune globulin by the cell involves the concept that the lymphocyte contains many "mini-genes" that exist in an orderly manner on its chromosomes. The lymphocytes that participate in the immune system can be identified as B and T cells. The B cell is one that has matured in the bursa or bone marrow and the T cell is one that matured in the thymus gland. They play different roles in the immune mechanism, as shown in Fig. 9.2 and as described below.

T cells are the most abundant type of circulating lymphocytes in adults. In order for an antigen to be recognized by a T cell, the antigen must first combine with a surface receptor on a presenting cell, such as a monocyte-macrophage cell. Special receptors on the T cell then recognize the surface-bound antigen, thereby activating the cell to produce antibodies and to produce two types of regulatory T cells known as "helper" and "suppressor" cells. These helper and suppressor cells are important in the immune systems since they function, respectively, to increase or to decrease normal antibody production by B cells as well as T cells. In normal, healthy persons the relative numbers of these two types of cells are delicately balanced. Such T cell immunity can be passively transferred from an immune person to a naive person only through transfer of the blood cells.

In addition certain T cells possess cytotoxic properties and other T cells can be activated by bacterial antigens to form cytotoxic T cells. They are so named because they can directly destroy invaders such as bacteria, fungi, and viruses and even some tumor cells. An additional function of antigen-activated T cells is their ability to induce other cells to release several mediators, such as lymphokines, which attract a variety of cells to inflammation sites in the body.

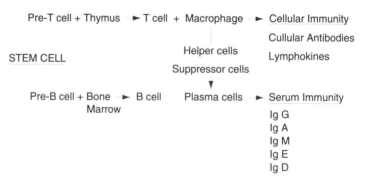

FIGURE 9.2   Source and role of B and T lymphocytes in the immune system. Modified from *Allergy Theory and Practice,* 2nd ed. (P. E. Korenblat and H. J. Wedner, Eds.), W.B. Saunders, Philadelphia, 1992.

About 25% of all peripheral blood lymphocytes in adults are B cells. When a B cell encounters a chemical antigen that fits the cell receptor, even if the affinity is weak, activation of a minigene leads to the production of antibody. Once this process begins, the cell will undergo point mutation of the immunoglobulin genes resulting in additional lymphocyte clones with greater and greater affinity for the initial hapten. Even if there is no further exposure to the hapten the new clones of lymphocytes remain in the circulation in a resting state, alert to any further exposure to the hapten.

Following the initial recognition of an antigen by B cells, a cascade of helper (and suppressor) cells mentioned above assist (or inhibit) the activated B cells to enlarge, divide, and develop antibody-secreting capability. At this time they become known as plasma cells. The antibodies that are produced appear in the serum where they are recognized in the gamma globulin fraction as IgG, IgA, IgM, IgE, and IgD globulins. B cell immunity can be passively transferred to a naive person via blood plasma. The entire system can produce numerous variations in immunoglobulin molecules and it is self-controlled by feedback-inhibitory mechanisms. It has been said that a mouse weighing less than 1 oz can make over 100 million different antibodies.

SUBSEQUENT EXPOSURE TO HAPTENS—THE ALLERGIC REACTION

After it was demonstrated that certain types of sensitization could be transferred to a naive person via the serum, it was found that the IgE protein was the responsible immunoglobulin. In the sensitized person reintroduction of the antigen allows for the reaction to take place between the antigen and the preformed circulating antibody. This complex then reacts with receptors on the mast cells and on basophils, causing them to release several "mediators" from their secretory granules into the extracellular environment. These mediators are pharmacologically active agents. Table 9.1 is a list of these mediators and their pharmacologic effects. The biologic effects of the mediators on the body constitute one form of allergic response or sensitization response.

THE IMMUNE MECHANISM IN TOXICOLOGY

The immunogenic mechanisms play a significant role in all branches of human health. These mechanisms are of particular importance in toxicology because so many simple chemicals have varying degrees of haptenic activity.

TABLE 9.1 Mediators and Biologic Effects of Immediate "Sensitization Reactions"[a]

Mediator	Effects
Intraglandular	
Histamine	Vasodilation, increased vasopermeability, pruritus, bronchoconstriction
Proteases (tryptase, chymase)	Degradation of blood vessel basement membranes, generation of vasoactive complement
Heparin	Complexes with proteases, inhibition of blood coagulation
ECF-A	Eosinophil chemotaxis
Neutrophil chemotactic factor	Neutrophil chemotaxis
Membrane-derived	
Prostaglandin D-2	Vasopermeability, bronchoconstriction
Leukotrienes	Vasopermeability, bronchoconstriction
Platelet-activating factor	Platelet aggregation, vasopermeability, bronchoconstriction, chemotaxis

[a] Modified from *Mediators of Immediate Hypersensitivity Reactions* (Serafin, W. E. and Austen, K. F.), *N. E. J. Med.* No. 1 1987. pp. 30–34.

The fact that simple chemical compounds can activate the immune system was first demonstrated by Landsteiner and co-workers (Landsteiner, J., and Jacobs, J., *J. Exp. Med.* **61:** 643, 1935, and *J. Exp. Med.* **64:** 625, 1936). Their observations have been confirmed and extended. These workers showed that certain dinitrobenzene derivatives could be injected or applied at frequent intervals and in amounts that would not produce an undesirable effect on the animal, and that after a lapse of 7 to 14 days, a subsequent injection or application of the same or a closely related compound would induce a tissue response at the site of application or systematically in the animal. They showed that certain derivatives of the dinitrobenzene nucleus were highly effective in initiating this response, whereas other derivatives of the same nucleus were essentially ineffective.

Those compounds that were capable of initiating the sensitizing phenomena contained halogenated radicals. If the halogen in the dinitrobenzene nucleus was replaced with a hydrogen, hydroxyl, methane, or amino group, the resultant compound was essentially nonsensitizing and nonreactive. Landsteiner theorized that the presence of the halogen facilitated stable binding of the simple chemical with an endogenous protein carrier, and this complex was the antigen that was capable of eliciting the formation of antibodies in the animal.

Many simple chemicals have haptenic qualities, and all degrees of such activity are found. For example, phenol is rarely antigenic, even under laboratory experimental conditions, whereas the sedative drug phethenylate (phenylethylhydantoin) induces allergic symptoms in virtually every human who receives the drug on multiple occasions. Certain chemical groupings appear to have the quality of conferring haptenic properties on the chemical. In a similar manner, certain radicals on specific amino acids are probably involved in the formation of the hapten–protein complex. A series of chemical groupings on the hapten and on the protein which would be expected to confer such activity has been compiled by Davies with the help of O-Mant and is reproduced in Table 9.2. The hapten–protein complex involves a firm binding mechanism which is almost certainly a covalent bonding mechanism that causes the loss of the chemical characteristics of both the hapten and the protein. Chemicals that react with protein in a readily reversible reaction (as by ionic binding or by Van der Waal's forces) probably do not form antigens.

Many chemicals do not appear to react with protein *in vitro,* but are known to be sensitizers (or haptens) in the intact animal. Such chemicals are believed to undergo metabolic alteration *in vivo,* yielding products that have haptenic properties. If a biotransformation product of a chemical is highly reactive with protein, chemicals that undergo similar metabolic

TABLE 9.2   Some Reactive Groups on Haptens and on Amino Acids Which Are Cabable of Reacting in the Formation of Antigens[a]

On hapten		On amino acid	
Diazonium	$-\overset{+}{N}=N$	Serine	$-OH$
Thiol	$-SH$	Lysine	$-NH_2$
Sulfonic acid	$-SO_3H$	Arginine	$-NHC-NH_2$ $\overset{\|}{NH}$
Aldehyde	$-CHO$		
		Cysteine	$-SH$
Quinone	$O = \langle\ \rangle = O$		
Active halogen		Cystine	$-S-S-$
		Tyrosine	$-\langle\ \rangle-OH$

[a] Data from Davies, G. E., *Proc. Eur. Soc. Study Drug Tox.* **4:**198, 1964.

transformation may be responsible for the formation of a hapten common to all chemicals in that group. Regardless of whether the chemical is the hapten, closely related compounds may effectively substitute for each other in the role of acting as a specific hapten. It is now generally accepted that there are some specific reactive groups on haptens and on amino acids that are capable of interaction leading to the formation of antigens. Table 9.2 lists some of these groups.

The formation of the antibody is dose-dependent with regard to the antigen. When antibodies are demonstrated in the plasma, they appear only after a latent period following initial administration of the hapten or precursor of the hapten. This is followed in succession by a log phase period of exponential rise in the antibody concentration (or titre) of the blood, a secondary stationary phase when the antibody concentration remains constant, and a subsequent decay period in antibody concentration. If a challenging dose of a sensitizing chemical is administered at a time when the antibody concentration is high, the immune response would be expected to be more extensive than it would be if the sensitizing chemical were administered when the antibody titre was low. Therefore, a challenging dose of a sensitizing chemical may or may not elicit an immune response, depending on the time of the administration of the challenging agent and the level of the antibody titre at that time.

Various serologic methods have been used to demonstrate the presence of circulating antibodies. Such tests are only infrequently successful in evaluating the presence or level of chemical-induced antibodies, although challenging doses of the chemical administered to the intact animal will produce the characteristic immune reactions in sensitized animals. Although several serologic tests (passive hemagglutination, complement fixation, and passive cutaneous anaphylaxis) have low limits of sensitivity, it is probable that antibodies can be present, but the number may be below levels detectable by these testing procedures.

Penicillin preparations are commonly a cause of sensitization in humans, and a brief discussion of these preparations demonstrates some of the complexities of the sensitization process. The penicillin molecule is generally believed to be incapable of acting as a hapten because of its low order of reactivity and the reversible nature of its reactivity with proteins. Therefore, the hapten is assumed to be either a biotransformation product of penicillin or a contaminant that is common to all preparations of penicillin. The assumption that a breakdown product is the responsible agent has some experimental support.

Although several breakdown products from penicillin are possible haptens, a breakdown product that seems to be involved is penicillinic acid. It is a normal contaminant of all penicillin preparations, it appears as an early degradation product of penicillin, and it is capable of reacting covalently with disulfide, sulfhydryl, or amide linkages. If penicillinic acid is reacted with an amino group at neutral pH, a penicilloyl linkage is formed. The reactions involved in the formation of the penicilloyl conjugate are shown in Fig. 9.3. Such a penicilloyl protein is highly antigenic in rabbits and guinea pigs. The antibodies that are formed can be detected in the serum and can be passively transferred to other animals. Furthermore, antipenicilloyl antibodies have been found in the serum of humans with a history of allergic reaction to penicillin. Although the penicilloyl group appears to be present in sensitization to penicillin, total allergy to penicillin probably involves multiple factors that characterize the genetic and immunologic status of the host.

In experimental toxicology, following the initial sensitizing dose of a chemical any subsequent doses are referred to as "challenge doses" which attempt to elicit the allergic or immune response. The antigen–antibody reaction is frequently a highly specific reaction in which only the specific antigen or hapten that was used for sensitization reacts with the antibody. Conversely, it may be stated that the antibody frequently will react only with the hapten or hapten–protein complex (antigen) that was used for sensitization. This mechanism is therefore utilized in protein immunochemistry for analytic purposes. However, the antigen–antibody reaction is not

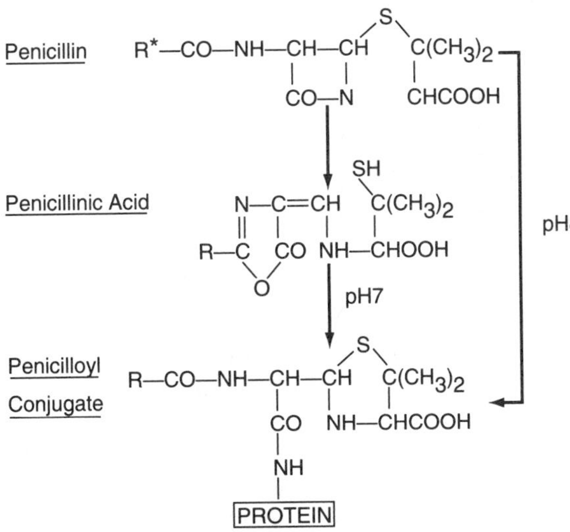

FIGURE 9.3   *R varies with the type of penicillin. From DeWeck, A. L., *Proc. Eur. Soc. Study Drug Tox.* **4:** 206, 1964.

always entirely specific for the hapten when simple chemicals are used to induce the formation of the antibody. For example, when a certain dinitrophenyl derivative acts as the hapten, the antibody produced against that hapten also reacts when other dinitrophenyl derivatives are used as the challenge dose, although the reaction is of lesser intensity than that produced by the hapten used to induce the antibody.

Because of the lack of absolute specificity in hapten–antibody reactions, the term "cross-sensitization" has developed to indicate this lack of specificity for simple chemical haptens. Cross-sensitization essentially means that an induced antibody may react with antigens formed from haptens of similar chemical structures. This concept is of considerable importance in immune reactions to xenobiotic chemicals and particularly to drugs. Many series of drugs have been developed, such as the barbiturates, the synthetic narcotics, and the sulfonamides, in which members of the series have similar pharmacologic actions, have similar structures, and are similarly biotransformed by the animal. Thus one member of a series may serve to sensitize an animal so that the immune response will occur when the animal is challenged with other members of the series of drugs. The phenomenon of cross-sensitization has been observed clinically between benzoic acid, *o*-hydroxybenzoic acid, *m*-hydroxybenzoic acid, and *p*-hydroxybenzoic acid esters. This is a particularly important cross-sensitization group of chemicals because of the extensive use of these esters as preservatives in nutrients, cosmetics, soaps, and drug preparations. Although cross-sensitization is generally considered to be limited to compounds having similar chemical structure, the similarity may not be obvious since cross-sensitization has been observed between the antibacterial agents neomycin and bacitracin, which represent distinctly different structures.

IMMUNE MECHANISMS IN CLINICAL TOXICOLOGY

In clinical medicine four types of immunologic responses are recognized. These are:

Type 1 (immediate responses). Humoral serum antibodies release pharmacologic agents from mast cells and basophils. An example is allergic rhinitis (hay fever).

Type 2 (cytotoxic responses). Compliment is involved and the antibodies are on the surface of cell membranes. The response by which body cells are killed may be very specific. An example is penicillin-induced anemia.

Type 3 (immune complex sensitization responses). Soluble antigen combines with antibodies in the serum yielding an immune complex; serum compliment is activated and the complex is deposited in specific tissues. An example is incompatible serum sickness.

Type 4 (delayed sensitization responses). Antigen-activated T cells suppress microbial infection mainly through macrophage activity and in the process enzymes may be released from the macrophages and lymphocytes. The enzymes destroy normal tissue cells. The process involves a 1- to 2-day delay before the tissue response is clinically manifested. Examples are contact dermatitis and the tuberculin reaction.

Types 1 through 3 can be transferred in the serum from sensitized to naive persons, whereas type 4 can only be transferred via the cells and the circulating antibody does not seem to be required.

The difficulties encountered in proving that a chemical is a cause of a toxic reaction, besides proving that the toxicity is due to a sensitization reaction in humans, are great unless the occurrence is so frequent that the cause–effect relationship becomes obvious. Current belief holds that whereas many of the adverse and abnormal reactions to chemicals are reported as sensitization reactions, proof of this is lacking. Compilations of adverse drug reactions, such as the Registry of Blood Dyscrasias of the American Medical Association, are useful to the practicing physician and lead to recognition of drugs commonly encountered in drug toxicities, but are of little value from the standpoint of shedding light on the mechanism involved in the production of the toxicity. However, by use of special methods, immune-mediated responses in the skin can be differentiated from simple irritant responses, thereby improving the evaluation of causation. Table 9.3 lists some classes and examples of materials that produce immunologic contact urticaria that have been seen in dermatology clinics.

A variety of chemicals are known to produce undesirable reactions in the skin of man when the skin is exposed to sunlight and, in some cases, to artificial light. These dermatologic lesions vary from sunburn-like responses to edematous, vesiculated, or bullous types of lesions. Since both exposure to light and the presence of the drug are involved, such reactions are called "photosensitivity" reactions. Two mechanisms are believed to be responsible for the reactions. The first is the phototoxic type, which is the result of a nonimmune mechanism and occurs on the first occasion of exposure to the drug plus light. By this mechanism the compound, which is present in the skin, absorbs energy (from the ultraviolet range of 2800 to 4000 Å) which converts the compound to a higher energy active state. The absorbed energy is reemitted as radiation energy, which becomes part of a photochemical reaction leading to cellular damage. Examples of compounds that are known to produce such phototoxic reactions are the

TABLE 9.3   A Selected List of Classes and Examples of Agents Producing Immunologic Contact Urticaria[a]

Class	Examples
Animal products	Blood, hair, silk, wool
Food	
Dairy	Cheese, milk
Fruits	Apple, orange, peach
Grains	Flour, wheat bran
Nuts	Peanut butter, sunflower seeds
Meats	Beef, chicken, lamb
Seafood	Fish, shrimp
Vegetables	Cabbage, onion, tomato
Fragrances & flavorings	Menthol, vanillin
Medicaments	Aspirin, penicillin, local anesthetics
Metals	Copper, nickel
Plant products	Perfumes, spices, rubber latex
Preservatives	Benzoic acid, parabens
Resins	Epoxy resin, formaldehyde resin

[a] Data from *Occupational and Industrial Dermatology* (H. I. Maiback, Ed.), 2nd ed., Year Book Publishers, Chicago, 1987.

coal tar derivatives pyridine and anthracene, the antibacterial agents dimethylchlortetracycline and sulfonamides, and the tranquilizer chlorpromazine.

The second type of photosensitive response to chemicals involves the haptene-allergic mechanism. The chemical or its metabolic product acts as the haptene, which combines with a tissue protein leading to the formation of an antigen which in turn elicits the formation of antibodies. On reexposure to the chemical plus exposure to light (electromagnetic energy of the proper wavelengths) the antigen–antibody response is manifested as cellular damage in the skin. There is probably a genetic basis for susceptibility to this mechanism, since only a small percentage of the population shows this form of photosensitivity to chemicals. Examples of agents that have been shown to induce this type of response are the thiazides, aminobenzoic acid, griseofulvin, promethazine, and chlorpropamide.

The cutaneous sensitization responses to chemicals have several common features which are summarized as follows: chemicals may be well tolerated for days, months, or years and suddenly give rise to sensitization reactions, and the sensitization response is different from the pharmacologic response. Chemicals that give different pharmacologic effects may give rise to identical allergic responses. The dosage necessary to produce the sensitization reaction is less than that required to produce the expected pharmacologic effect. Once a reaction has occurred, it will recur regularly on administration of the chemical, even in small doses. A chemical may produce a different sensitization response in different persons as well as in the same person at different times.

The intensity and nature of an allergic reaction may be of such minor toxicologic importance that it is of little significance. In some cases, continued exposure to the offending chemical will be accompanied by gradual disappearance of the allergic response. However, all sensitization reactions are related to the dose of the challenging agent, to the antibody titre, and to the route of administration of the chemical. In the absence of knowledge of the antibody titre, administration of drugs or chemicals to known sensitized persons or animals may result in severe sensitization reactions. Such a procedure should be approached with extreme caution. The nature of the sensitization response is not always predictable. On one occasion or in one person, the response may be manifested as a cutaneous reaction, in another it may be a vascular response, and in a third it may be a blood cell suppression response.

ACTIVATION AND SUPPRESSION OF THE IMMUNE SYSTEM

Failure of the immune system does occur clinically when there are deficient amounts or activity of various components of the system. Examples are diseases produced by compliment deficiency, phagocytic cell defects, lymphocyte deficiency, and particularly B or T cell deficiency. In recent years because of the worldwide awareness of Acquired Immunodeficiency Syndrome (AIDS), interest in methods of improving the overall activity of the immune systems has achieved a very high priority. Basically, AIDS is caused by infection with Human Immunodeficiency Virus (HIV) with a resulting decrease in the total number of lymphocytes and a disproportionate decrease in the absolute number of specific T cells. Currently there is no antiviral drug that will cure AIDS. In those immune deficiencies that involve antibody deficiency, antibodies can be replaced by treatment with intravenous serum globulin preparations, and purified IgG, IgA, and IgM are also available. In severe combined immunodeficiency disease, bone marrow transplantation has been used. As far as immune deficiency to xenobiotics is concerned, it might even be viewed as a beneficial condition were it not for the fact that the same system would fail to achieve its main function of protecting against microbial infection.

Interest in suppression of the immune mechanism has been widespread because of the role of this mechanism in allergy and autoimmune disease in humans and in rejection of foreign grafts in transplantation experiments, and because it is basically involved with cell proliferation mechanisms in the animal. Whereas there is no agent that will selectively suppress only the antibody-forming mechanism, any procedure or drug that suppresses cell proliferation or interferes with protein or nucleic acid formation will, under proper experimental conditions, suppress the antibody-forming mechanism.

Clinical allergists commonly use an approach to treat allergy called Allergy Immunotherapy. The procedure has been used for many years in patients that have allergic rhinitis (hay fever). The procedure is to treat the patient once or twice weekly with subcutaneous injections of the antigen, using as the initial dose one that has been shown to be tolerated by skin tests. Subsequent doses may be increased depending on the occurrence of reactions to the lower dose. A precise explanation for the claimed effectiveness of allergy immunotherapy has not been demonstrated but the apparent goal of the procedure is twofold. One purpose is to attempt to produce a blocking antibody which can effectively compete with the existing antibody for the antigen. Second, the procedure is helpful in producing a tolerance type of response, presumably by decreasing the sensitivity of the target cells to the antigen–antibody response. It is known that when adult animals are given repeated subimmunogenic doses of an antigen, or when they are given excessively high doses of the purified antigen, this leads to the development of a tolerance that is characterized by suppression of the immune response to the particular antigen when it is subsequently administered in what is normally an immunogenic form. The mechanism of this tolerance induction is not known, but it is believed to be associated with an inhibition of lymphoid cell formation.

The effect of irradiation on the immune response has been shown to be either activating or depressing to the mechanism. Generally irradiation will be maximally depressing if the animals are irradiated a few hours to 2 days before sensitization with the antigen. However, the opposite effect of activation of mild sensitization in immune disease may follow whole-body radiation. Similar observations have been made in regard to the effects of chemical agents on the immune mechanism. Chemicals of interest in this regard are generally those that are powerful inhibitors of cellular proliferation and differentiation. Examples are alkylating agents such as mustards (methyl-bis-beta chlorethylamine or tris-beta chlorethylamine), purine and pyrimidine analogs such as 6-mercaptopurine and thioguanine, and antibiotics such as Actinomycin D. Whereas these agents are generally considered as nonspecific suppressive compounds, their effects on immune mechanisms largely depend on the experimental design used in the test, the species studied, and timing of administration.

The sensitization reaction represents an insidious form of chemical-induced toxicity. Persons who have a history of intolerance to certain foods or chemicals, especially drugs, or who have a history of allergic disease such as hay fever or asthma should be given drugs with caution. There is no definitive manner by which sensitization to a chemical can be predicted in specific individuals. A person should not be exposed to a known sensitizing chemical either in the form of a drug or in the process of occupational endeavor unless the benefits of such exposure outweigh the potential hazard associated with such exposure. Once the process of sensitization has occurred, it is more reasonable to expect that the person will continue to be sensitized for an indefinite period of time than to expect that desensitization can be accomplished or will spontaneously occur in time. It is not reasonable to use drugs that are known sensitizers (such as the antibiotics) in minor illness when such drugs may be desired and necessary for life-saving purposes on some subsequent occasion.

CHAPTER **10**

The Basis of Selective Toxicity

$\mathbf{S}$elective toxicity refers to the variability in toxicologic response of cells to xenobiotic agents. Although there are excellent examples of variation in response of different members of the plant kingdom to chemicals, the discussion here will be concerned only with variation between biologic cells, tissues, and organisms when they are exposed to foreign chemicals.

Biologic variation between cells is frequently observed as a variation between whole animals, and much of this text has been directed toward a description of some mechanisms that account for variation between animals in response to chemicals. Most chemicals that serve a useful purpose for man do so by influencing the function of only a very limited number or type of cells or systems. That is, the xenobiotic agent affects a normal biochemical system and interferes with the functions that are normally accomplished by that system. When a xenobiotic agent reacts at some specific biochemical site, that site is commonly referred to as the "target" or "receptor" for the agent(s). Cells that do not possess the proper receptor would not be affected in the same manner as those that do possess the receptor. Although there are many complex factors involved in the xenobiotic–receptor interaction, the system involves at least two basic requirements in order for a xenobiotic agent to be selectively active on one cell and not on another. One requirement is that it (or a biotransformation product) must gain access to the cell. Second, the cell must contain a receptor for the agent. Consequently the mechanisms involved in selective toxicity are those that influence the concentration (i.e., translocation systems) and chemical properties of the agent and its products (i.e., biotransformation systems) and the existence of specific receptor systems in cells. These mechanisms are shown in Table 10.1. The following text presents some examples of each.

SELECTIVE TOXICITY DUE TO
TRANSLOCATION MECHANISMS

In the intact animal, whenever a mechanism exists that is able to concentrate (bioaccumulate) a xenobiotic agent, the result is an elevated probability of occurrence of toxicity at that site. For example, in mammals the kidney functions as an excretory organ that is capable of excreting products from the blood via the urine at elevated concentrations. One example whereby this mechanism enables a compound to become selectively toxic to kidney cells is the case of uranium bicarbonate. This compound is water soluble and is readily excreted from the blood. The kidney returns the bicarbonate ions and water to the blood and retains the uranyl ions which are concentrated as the urine is being formed. This biocentration of uranyl ions takes place in the tubules of the excretory units of the kidney and concentrations are reached that produce selective renal tubular cell damage.

Barriers to absorption or translocation of a chemical may be present in some species of animals and not in others, thereby influencing concentrations of a chemical in different species. Studies by the author which were concerned with the toxicity of *N,N'*-Bis-(3 methanesulfonyloxypropionyl)-1,2-propanediamine, an anticancer agent, have shown that dogs that received 10 mg/kg of this compound per day, either by mouth, mixed with feed, or by the intravenous route, showed severe depression of white blood cell formation at the end of 5 days. Rats or monkeys tolerated 100 to 500 mg/kg per day by mouth, mixed with feed, for 1 to 3 months without effect on the white blood cells. It was subsequently shown that the drug was not destroyed by admixing it with the feed used for the rats or

TABLE 10.1 Mechanisms of Selective Toxicity

A. Mechanisms involving alteration of available effective concentration of the chemical at effector sites
   1. Due to translocation factors
   2. Due to biotransformation mechanisms
B. Mechanisms involving the presence or absence of target systems susceptible to the chemical

monkeys. (The same rats or rhesus monkeys subsequently received 10 mg/kg of the compound per day for 5 days by intravenous administration and showed the same toxic effect on blood cells as was shown in the dog.) Thus, selective toxicity to chemicals between species can be the result of variations in absorption or translocation processes.

The cyclic chlorinated insecticide chlorphenothane (DDT) owes its effectiveness on the insect at least partly to the fact that it is readily absorbed directly through the chitinous exoskeleton of the insect. DDT is only poorly absorbed through the skin of mammals. However, it has already been mentioned that because insects are small compared to mammals, they have a greater body surface area in relation to weight than do mammals. Therefore, in an atmosphere of DDT, insects receive a greater dose through the skin in relation to body weight than do mammals, thereby making an apparent selective action of DDT on insects the result of both high dose and ineffective barrier mechanisms in the insect.

Another interesting and important example of the effect of altered translocation of compounds as a mechanism of selective toxicity is demonstrated by fluoride and particularly fluoroacetate-induced toxicity. For many years it was believed that fluoroacetate produced its toxicity by competing with citrate for active sites on the enzyme aconitase, thereby blocking the citric acid cycle. As shown in Fig. 10.1 carbohydrate and fat serve as fuel, through conversion to acetyl-CoA, for the energy processes of the citric acid cycle. The cycle serves as a machine for the metabolism of acetyl-CoA. In the

DIAGRAMMATIC REPRESENTATION OF THE
MECHANISM OF FLUOROACETATE-INDUCED TOXICITY

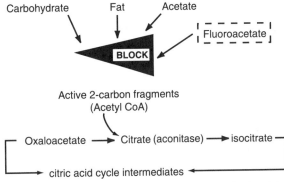

FIGURE 10.1   Transfer of acetate through membranes in the mitochondrial system of the cell is mediated by a carrier system which is blocked by fluoroacetate, thereby depleting the fuel source for the citric acid cycle.

cycle, citrate is converted to isocitrate by the enzyme aconitase. Blockage of this enzyme by fluoroacetate is one mechanism by which the citric acid cycle would be blocked. However, the enzymes of the citric acid cycle are located in membranous bound structures in the cell known as the mitochondria. There is now evidence that the action of fluoroacetate may be to complex with and inactivate a carrier substance that functions primarily to transfer acetate into the mitochondria. Therefore an important action of fluoroacetate may be to competitively block translocation of specific nutrients within the cell.

SELECTIVE TOXICITY DUE TO
BIOTRANSFORMATION MECHANISMS

The processes of biotransformation supply a mechanism that accounts for many examples of selective toxicity. Since biotransformation may result in destruction of the biologically active form of a chemical or formation of a more toxic product, it is apparent that the presence or absence of such mechanisms within members of a species will effectively alter the concentration of the parent chemical in the biologic specimen. If the biotransformation process involves detoxication of the parent chemical, a failure or absence of the process may induce toxicity by failing to terminate the drug action. Examples of such a selective toxicity induced by genetic deviations between members of a species are described in Chapter 6.

In contrast to the examples of genetic deviations in biotransformation mechanisms within a species, such mechanisms may be present or absent in different species or strains, thereby accounting for strain or species selectivity in chemical-induced toxicity. In this manner certain strains of bacteria, particularly gram-negative bacilli, are resistant to penicillin at least partly because they elaborate an enzyme (penicillinase) which inactivates penicillin. Some strains of houseflies and mosquitoes are resistant to the insecticide malathion by virtue of their ability to produce a specific enzyme (esterase) that inactivates malathion.

The relative rates of activation and inactivation of a xenobiotic are of great importance in determining their overall biologic effect. The following example demonstrates how this can contribute to a selective toxic action of organophosphates on insects. The organophosphates produce toxicity primarily by their ability to inhibit the enzyme acetylcholinesterase (AChE). Two types of such organic phosphates are the direct inhibitors of AChE and the indirect inhibitors of AChE. The direct inhibitors, such as diisopropyl fluorophosphate and methylisopropyl phosphonofluoridate, do not require metabolic conversion (oxidation) to active forms, whereas the indirect inhibitors such as Parathion or Malathion are metabolically activated (oxidized by microsomal enzymes) to compounds that are able to inactivate AChE more rapidly. The activated derivatives are then hydrolyzed (by other esterases) and are thereby eventually inactivated. Basically, a species that could activate the indirect type of inhibitor but could not hydrolyze it would accumulate the active form, and thereby would be susceptible to the toxic effects of the compound. In contrast to this a species which could hydrolyze the indirectly acting organic phosphate instead of activating it would be expected to be resistant to the action of the compound. Different species of biologic specimens carry on these activation (oxidation) and inactivation (hydrolysis) reactions at different rates, thereby creating a condition in which the balance between these reaction rates determines the effective concentrations of the active forms and the extent of toxic effect of the organic phosphate in the species under study.

Figure 10.2 shows these reactions in the case of Malathion and the relative rates of the reactions in insects and mammals. Mammals hydrolyze and thereby rapidly inactivate Malathion, thus reducing the quantity available for conversion to Malaoxon, which is readily hydrolyzed to inactive products. Since insects do not as readily hydrolyze Malathion, more of it is available for oxidation to Malaoxon, which is more stable in the insect than in the mammal. With doses of Malathion being equal in the two species, therefore, enzyme activity would result in a greater accumulation of the active oxygen analog in the insect than in the mammal, thereby contributing to the selectively toxic action on the insect.

The foregoing examples collectively represent mechanisms that alter the available concentration of a chemical in an animal or at specific sites in

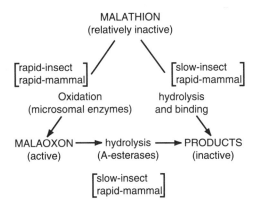

FIGURE 10.2 Pathways for biotransformation of the organic phosphate insecticide Malathion, and the relative rates of the reactions in insects and mammals.

the animal in comparison to the concentration of the compound that may be present in other tissues or other species of animals. In this sense, these mechanisms collectively represent a single type of selective toxicity of chemicals.

SELECTIVE TOXICITY DUE TO THE PRESENCE OR ABSENCE OF RECEPTORS

The second mechanism involved in selective pharmacologic or toxicologic action of chemicals on cells involves the existence or absence of specific targets or receptor systems in the exposed cells (Table 10.1). In this case, the concentration of the compound to which various cells are exposed is the same for all cells, but only certain cells are affected. The selective action of the normal neurohumors and endocrine substances, as well as that of many drugs, involves this mechanism. When administered to mammals, acetylcholine or norepinephrine, which are normal neurohumors liberated at the ends of nerves, selectively react only at specific sites on membranes that are presumed to contain specific receptors only for one or the other of these agents, but not for both. In fact, the specificity of the receptor may be so selective that only one isomeric form of a compound will react to any significant extent with that receptor. The adrenergic amines l-epinephrine and d-epinephrine are examples of this selective action of optical isomers; the levo isomer has 20 times the activity of the dextro isomer.

For our purposes it is not necessary to go into the details of receptor theory, but it is necessary to recognize that many of the most potent toxic agents known to man produce their biologic effects by reacting with chemicals (receptors) that are involved with normal essential biologic mechanism(s) with a resultant blockade of the mechanism(s). For example, cyanide and azide block oxidative cell metabolism, d-tubocurarine blocks transmission of nerve impulses to skeletal muscle, and botulinum toxin blocks release of the neurotransmitter at the nerve–muscle junction. Some rodenticides are useful because they show species-selective action due to the presence of receptors in rodents which are not present in man. An example is norbormide, which acts on receptors in smooth muscle in rats that are not present in man, dogs, or cats. The result is that doses of norbormide that are lethal to the rat are nontoxic to the other species.

Many biochemical enzymatic reactions are selectively specific with regard to the substrates that may be utilized in the reaction. In fact, such reactions are similar to the chemical-receptor types of reactions and also may be stereo-specific, that is, only one optical isomer is utilized or synthesized in the reaction. An example is the action of arginase, which effects hydrolysis of only the levo form of arginine. Other enzymatic systems may have only group specificity and will utilize only substrates that are closely related chemically; an example is the enzyme acetylcholinesterase, which hydrolyzes not only acetylcholine, but also acetyl-β-methylcholine and triacetin. Still other enzyme systems in the mammal have a very low specificity of action, an example being the lipases, which hydrolyze most fats.

Many drugs have as the basis for their selectivity of action the fact that chemically they are sufficiently similar to normal enzyme substrates to permit them to compete with or displace the normal substrates for the active sites on enzyme systems in the animal. It is believed that if the drug has a sufficient affinity for reaction with the active groups of the enzyme, it occupies the active sites on the enzyme in much the same manner that the normal substrate occupies the same sites on the enzyme. Although the drug may act to occupy the active sites on the enzyme, usually the drug is at best a poor substrate and may simply occupy the active sites on the enzyme so that they are no longer available for the natural substrate. The result is inhibition of the enzyme. If the enzyme is part of an essential chain of enzymatic reactions necessary to produce a biologic response, that physiological mechanism is blocked. The blockade may be due to competition between the drug and the normal substrate for the active sites on the enzyme, in which case the drug can be displaced from the enzyme simply by increasing the concentration of the normal substrate.

A good example of a competitive inhibition mechanism which is responsible for selectivity of the action of a chemical is shown by the antibacterial sulfonamide drugs. Almost 60 years ago it was shown that p-aminobenzoic acid (PABA) would competitively prevent the lethal action of sulfonamide on susceptible strains of bacteria. Many subsequent investigations regarding the mechanism of this competitive action between PABA and sulfonamide drugs have led to the conclusion that PABA is essential for the formation of one or more coenzymes of which folic acid is an essential component. These coenzymes play an important role in conversion of amino acids and in the formation of purines. PABA therefore appears to be an essential "nutrient" in those bacteria that cannot utilize preformed folic acid in the media in which they are grown but must synthesize their own folic acid. PABA is not essential in those strains of bacteria that are capable of utilizing preformed folic acid from the media in which they are grown. This accounts for the selectivity of lethal action of sulfonamide drugs for specific strains of bacterial organisms that are not able to utilize preformed folic acid. The human uses performed folic acid and is therefore not susceptible to this action of the sulfonamide compounds.

An example of the competitive inhibition type of reaction in which the specific enzyme systems involved are not completely definable is the competition between vitamin K and Dicumarol. Vitamin K is essential for the formation of certain globulin proteins in the liver of most mammals. Dicumarol selectively competes with vitamin K in these reactions in the liver of mammals, thereby causing failure in the formation of the globulins. The action of Dicumarol on this system can be reversed if the concentration of available vitamin K is increased.

In contrast to the competitive enzymatic inhibition mechanism described above, the drug–substrate complex may involve strong covalent bonding forces so that the enzyme is virtually irreversibly inactivated. An example of an almost irreversible enzyme–drug complex is the reaction between the organic phosphates (such as methyl isopropyl phosphonofluoridate) and the enzyme acetylcholinesterase. The basis of action of these drugs is their selective effect on specific enzyme systems within a species, and their effect is predominantly on the cells or tissues containing that enzyme system. Basically, in these examples the enzyme (or active sites on the enzyme) act as receptors for the xenobiotic agent.

Similar mechanisms can account for selectivity between species. Certain antibiotic drugs owe their effectiveness on bacteria to the fact that they selectively act on a target system that is essential for either reproduction or maintenance of viability of the bacteria. The same target system is either nonexistent or nonessential in the physiology of mammals. For example, the lethal action of penicillin affects only actively multiplying bacterial cells. Penicillin interferes with the synthesis by the bacteria of mucopeptides and teichoic acid which are necessary, strength-supplying, structural components of the bacterial cell walls. Since the actively multiplying bacterial cells must maintain a high internal osmotic pressure compared to their external environment, penicillin-induced defective cell walls lead to bizarre and fragile forms and eventual death of the bacterial cells without affecting human cells.

The potential usefulness of selectively active chemicals on biologic mechanisms has progressed rapidly in the fields of agriculture and pharmacology, but is only in its infancy in the science of toxicology. It is evident that a prelude to the systematic development of selectively toxic substances is a better understanding of the biochemical systems that regulate and control the growth and viability of undesirable forms of cells. Such undesirable cells are manifested as cells in the liver that accumulate lipid or are replaced by fibrous tissue, cells that undergo degenerative changes without replacement, or cells that fail to maintain their state of differentiation and therefore become the malignant accumulations of undesirable cells. The evasive and complex nature of the biochemical mechanisms that initiate and control reproduction, differentiation, maturation, degeneration, and regeneration of cells may preclude early absolute chemical identification of the subtle differences between cells that may be subject to attack by selectively toxic chemicals. Perhaps one "key" lead regarding the nature of such a point of attack will enable rational systematic development of selectively toxic agents without chemical identification of the receptor or receptors involved.

CHAPTER **11**

The Basis of
Antidotal Therapy

In a situation in which a harmful effect of a chemical presents a threat to an economic species, it is necessary to be able either to reverse the harmful effect or at least to prevent further harm from the chemical. It is axiomatic that if a chemical causes death of living tissue, no procedure is successful in reversing such an effect on those cells, and new cells and tissues must be formed if the organ is to continue to function.

In contrast to this, a harmful effect of a chemical may consist of mild to severe impairment of function short of death of the biologic cells, tissues, or whole animal. Under this condition, procedures that are specifically directed toward limiting the intensity of the effect or reversing the effect are useful for preventing further harm. Such procedures are referred to as "antidotal procedures" or "antidotal therapy." When the use of a chemical is involved in such a procedure, the chemical is referred to as an "antidotal agent." Successful antidotal therapy becomes a necessity especially whenever humans are the economic species involved in harmful effects from chemicals. Therefore, most of the developments in antidotal therapy are concerned with protection of humans, or at least animals, from the toxic effects of chemicals.

GENERAL PRINCIPLES

All antidotal procedures are based on two concepts (see Chapters 2 and 3): first, that the intensity of all chemical–biologic reactions is related to the dose, or more accurately to the concentration, of the chemical at the effector sites in the tissue; second, following administration of a chemical to a biologic specimen, the concentration of the chemical within the tissues is dependent upon the ability of biologic barriers to prevent its translocation and on the chemical properties of the compound, which permit or prevent its translocation in the tissue.

Since translocation of a chemical is a time-dependent process, it may be said that the intensity of all chemical–biologic reactions is time-dependent. The following is an example of how these two concepts are concerned with antidotal procedures. In order for an animal to be exposed to a chemical, a route of administration must be involved. Any route of administration could be considered. If the intravenous or inhalation route is involved, the time intervals would be much shorter than for the oral route of administration, but the principle that time is involved in translocation of the chemical to effector sites would still be valid. For the purpose of presenting an example, the oral route is used here.

Following oral administration of an excessive dose of the chemical, depending on the chemical properties of the agent involved, it is absorbed or translocated to the blood from which it is in turn translocated to the various tissues of the animal. For practical purposes, the concentration of the chemical in the blood or in the tissues rises at a rate directly related to the dose and inversely related to the rate of termination (excretion, storage deposition, and metabolic transformation) of action of the chemical at the effector site in the animal. If it is assumed that the oral dose of the chemical is sufficient to produce a harmful effect, that effect will occur in relation to time when a toxic concentration of the chemical is present in the blood or at the effector site. Shown in Fig. 11.1A is the nature of the curve that would be achieved if an animal were given a selected compound in a dose that would produce a measurable toxic effect, but not death of the animal. It is apparent that if death of the animal occurred, the curve would terminate at that point in time. If death of the animal did not occur, at some point in time absorption of the chemical from the gastrointestinal tract would be complete, and the quantity of the chemical at the effector sites would decrease in direct relation to the rate of termination of action of the chemical at the effector sites. If the toxic effect consists of a reversible phenomenon, as the concentration of the chemical declines with the progression of time, recovery of the animal is complete. Any reversible tissue damage that may remain following termination of the existence of the

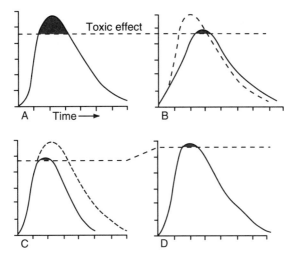

FIGURE 11.1   Schematic curves representing the relation between the effect in terms of concentration of a chemical at effector sites and time after oral ingestion of a hypothetical toxic chemical. See text for derivation of the curves.

chemical in the animal undergoes repair or regeneration in time, provided additional assault by the chemical is avoided. Tissue in which there is nonreversible, chemical-induced damage also undergoes replacement or fibrosis in time if the animal survives. Furthermore, the major difference between chemical-induced damage to tissue following acute exposure and that following chronic exposure to a chemical would be a difference in the time intervals involved for induction and recovery from the toxicity.

The curve in Fig. 11.1A contains a shaded portion which represents the area of time in relation to the intensity of effect when the toxic effect of the chemical is manifested in the animal. Since antidotal therapy is directed toward effectively abolishing the shaded area in the figure, there are three obvious procedures that would accomplish this objective: (1) decrease the slope of the rising portion of the curve, (2) increase the slope of the descending portion of the curve or displace the descending portion of the curve to the left, and (3) elevate the level or threshold at which the toxic range of effect occurs.

The effect of each of these three procedures on the shaded portion of the curve in Fig. 11.1A is shown, respectively, in Figs. 11.1B, 11.1C, and 11.1D. All three conditions constitute mechanisms that can be effectively utilized in antidotal procedures. The slope of the rising portion of the curve may be decreased (Fig. 11.1B) by actual or virtual removal of the unabsorbed portion of the chemical from the gastrointestinal tract or by removal of the chemical before it is translocated within the animal to the effector site. The slope of the descending portion of the curve (Fig. 11.1C) can be increased and moved to the left by increasing the rate of termination of action at the effector sites by increasing the rate of excretion of the compound via the kidney or lungs or by other physiological excretory mechanisms, by promoting the inactivation of the compound by chemically binding it to nonspecific effector sites, and by mechanically translocating the chemical to the exterior of the animal. Finally, the threshold at which the toxic effect occurs can be elevated (Fig. 11.1D) by the administration of antidotal chemicals that either directly or indirectly pharmacologically antagonize the toxic effect of the chemical, or by mechanical procedures which substitute for, or carry out, the function that is impaired by the toxic effect.

In actual practice in human clinical toxicology, each of the three possible mechanisms for influencing toxicity is accomplished either by nonspecific or by specific methods. The nonspecific methods are those general methods which are applicable to large numbers of chemicals (that is, nonspecified chemicals). The specific methods are used when the specific compounds that are the probable or potential cause of the toxicity have been identified. Table 11.1 categorizes the various nonspecific antidotal procedures that are available, as well as the specific procedures as they are used for altering the time–response curves shown in Fig. 11.1.

PROCEDURES FOR DECREASING ABSORPTION OR TRANSLOCATION

The antidotal procedures for limiting absorption on exposure to topically applied offending chemicals are mechanical removal and the use of chemical agents that will combine with and detoxify the offending chemical. Following the ingestion of an amount of an offending chemical that is potentially adequate to produce a toxic or harmful effect, antidotal therapy may involve one or more of several procedures. Removal of the chemical from the stomach, either by gastric lavage or by the use of an emetic, represents the most direct procedure for preventing absorption of the chemical.

Gastric lavage is accomplished by inserting a tube into the stomach and washing the stomach with water or any suitable and relatively harmless solvent for the agent involved. Water is the lavage fluid preferred since it is the most innocuous of fluids; however, it would not be as effective as other solvents for substances that are only slightly soluble in water. In the case of lipid-soluble agents, liquid petrolatum would be a suitable lavage agent. If other solvents are used, the potential toxicity of the solvent should be considered an added hazard to the procedure. Regardless of the solvent properties of water, the mechanical irrigation of the stomach with a water lavage would assist in removing particulate matter. The lavage procedure is practical only for removal of material that is in the stomach and does not remove material that has passed into the upper intestine.

An additional procedure for actual removal of the stomach contents is through the use of emetic agents. In humans, emesis can be induced by parenteral injection of apomorphine or by oral administration of syrup of ipecac. Apomorphine-induced emesis may be severe and the emesis does not lead to elimination of the apomorphine, which is in the circulation. In contrast to this, emesis that is induced by ipecac is primarily a consequence of a local action of the ipecac on the stomach, and the emesis results in the elimination of not only the potentially toxic agent, but also at least a portion of the ipecac. For this reason, ipecac would be the emetic of choice whenever an emetic agent is indicated in an antidotal procedure. Both drugs have a latent period of approximately 5 to 15 min between their administration and the induction of vomiting.

Properly performed lavage or the use of emetics seem to be of about equal efficiency in emptying the stomach. The time interval after the ingestion by mouth of amounts of a substance that would be potentially harmful is a very important factor to consider when emetics or lavage are to be used.

Animal studies suggest that when sedation is evident following ingestion of overdoses of sedative types of drugs, the production of emesis by emetic drugs cannot be relied on. That is, the sedative drug antagonizes the action of the emetic drug. If the intensity of sedation is so great that the subject is unconscious, the induction of vomiting is contraindicated unless particular caution is used to prevent aspiration of vomitus that may lodge in the subject's upper pharynx. In children who may have ingested petroleum products such as kerosene, it is a controversial subject regarding whether any attempts should be made to empty the stomach because of the high probability that some of the kerosene would be aspirated into the lungs with a resultant pneumonitis. On the other hand, it may be proper to use emetics or lavage if there is reason to believe that the child may suffer more serious toxicity than that of a pneumonitis if no stomach emptying procedure is used. Each case of potential clinical intoxication from ingestion of a chemical agent requires a general assessment of all factors involved before treatment is initiated. In any case, the treatment should not be more harmful to the patient than the absence of treatment. For example, strong salt (table salt, NaCl) solutions should not be used to induce vomiting because the procedure is not a reliable one and there is a great possibility of producing salt intoxication.

TABLE 11.1 Mechanisms and Examples in Antidotal Therapy

I. Decrease the ascending slope of the time–response curve
  A. By influencing the rate of absorption of material from the gastrointestinal tract
    1. Nonspecific methods
      a. Emetics (apomorphine, syrup of ipecac)
      b. Mechanical-induced emesis (finger in upper pharynx)
      c. Stomach lavage
      d. Chemical neutralization (acid–base neutralization)
      e. Adsorption (activated charcoal)
    2. Specific methods
      a. Formation of less toxic complex

Agent	Antidote	Product
Iron	Sod. bicarbonate	Ferrous carbonate
Iron	Desferroxamine	Chelated iron
Silver nitrate	Sod. Chloride	Silver Chloride
Strychnine	Pot. permanganate	Oxidation product
Nicotine	Pot. permanganate	Oxidation product
Fluoride	Calcium lactate	Calcium fluoride

  B. By influencing distribution or translocation of agent to receptor site
    1. Nonspecific methods
      a. Ion trapping by altering blood pH (may be used when therapy involves correcting acid–base balance)
      b. Substitute alternate binding sites (infusion of albumin)
    2. Specific methods
      a. Produce less toxic product, competitively block metabolic biotransformation

Agent	Antidote	Product or effect
Cyanide	Methemoglobin	Cyanmethemoglobin
Cyanide	Thiosulfate	Thiocyanate
Methanol	Ethanol	Competitive block
Fluoroacetate	Acetate or monoacetin	Competitive substitution
Heparin	Protamine	Complex formation

II. Increase the descending slope of the time–response curve
  A. By increasing the rate of elimination
    1. Nonspecific methods
      a. Hemodialysis
      b. Peritoneal dialysis
      c. Exchange transfusion
      d. Adjust pH and diuresis (alkalinize urine for weak organic acids and acidify urine for weak organic bases)
    2. Specific methods
      a. Enhance excretion or form less toxic product by chelation or complex formation

(continues)

TABLE 11.1 (*Continued*)

Agent	Antidote	Mechanism
Bromide ion	Chloride ion	Enhance renal excretion
Strontium, radium	Calcium	Enhance renal excretion
Lead, nickel, cobalt, copper	EDTA	Chelation
Mercury, arsenic, gold	BAL	Chelation
Copper	d-Penicillamine	Chelation
Botulinus toxin	Antitoxin	Complex
Organic phosphate	Pralidoxime	Nucleophilic enzyme reactivation
Acetaminophen	n-Acetylcysteine	Less toxic metabolite

III. Elevation of the threshold for toxicity in the time–response curve
   A. By clinical support of vital functions or the use of pharmacologic antagonistic agents
     1. Nonspecific methods
       a. Mechanical artificial respiration to maintain oxygenation of blood or hyperbaric oxygen
       b. Maintain circulation of blood (counter shock therapy, plasma expanders, vasoconstrictors)
       c. Maintain electrolyte balance
       d. Maintain renal function
     2. Specific methods
       a. Use of pharmacologic antagonists or alternate pathways

Agent	Antidote	Mechanism
Morphine	Naloxone	Antagonism
Carbon monoxide	Oxygen	Antagonism
Dicumarol, Warfarin	Vitamin K	Antagonism
Organophosphates	Atropine	Antagonism
Curare	Neostigmine	Antagonism
Methotrexate	Folinic acid	Alternate pathway
5-Fluorouracil	Thymidine	Alternate pathway
6-Mercaptopurine	Purine	Alternate pathway
Lysergic acid diethylamide	Phenothiazine	Antagonism

In addition to the actual physical removal of an offending chemical from the stomach, virtual removal may be accomplished by the use of substances that effectively react with, firmly bind with, or adsorb the offending chemical. When the identity of the offending chemical is known, specific agents may be administered orally for this purpose. Examples are the administration of chelating agents such as calcium ethylenediaminetetraacetic acid (CaNa$_2$–EDTA) for chelation of metals, or the administration of activated charcoal to adsorb a variety of compounds. Chemical neutralization or chelation results in detoxication of the offending chemical. The adsorbent property of activated charcoal varies considerably depending upon the agent to be adsorbed (Table 11.2). Adsorption is not the same as chemical destruction, since adsorption may lead to release of the offending chemical as the pH of the environment changes during passage of the material through the gastrointestinal tract. Regardless of these factors adsorption *in* the stomach of material that otherwise might be absorbed *from* the stomach results in a delay of translocation of the offending chemical.

The "universal antidote" (one part magnesium oxide, one part tannic acid, and two parts activated charcoal) has been used as a combination of agents to perform several functions, since magnesium oxide neutralizes acids without gas formation and tannic acid forms insoluble salts with certain alkaloids and metals. However, it has been shown that tannic acid or magnesium oxide interferes with the adsorbent activity of activated charcoal. It is also known that if tannic acid is permitted to be absorbed,

TABLE 11.2   **Amounts of Various Substances Adsorbed from Aqueous Solutions by 1 g of Activated Charcoal (Carbo. Med. Merck)**

Substance	Maximal adsorption (mg)
Mercuric chloride	1800
Sulfanilamide	1000
Strychnine nitrate	950
Morphine hydrochloride	800
Atropine sulfate	700
Nicotine	700
Barbital	700
Salicylic acid	550
Phenol	400
Phenobarbital sodium	300–350
Aprobarbital sodium	300–350
5,5-Diallyl barbital sodium	300–350
Hexobarbital sodium	300–350
Cyclobarbital calcium	300–350
Alcohol	300
Potassium cyanide	35

Note. Data from Gosselin and Smith, *Clin. Pharmacol. Ther.* **7:**282, 1966.

it is capable of producing liver toxicity in some species of animals. Thus, it would seem that the mixture of agents used in the "universal antidote" defeats the purpose of attempting to achieve a universal effect by combining several antidotal agents in one preparation, and exposes the animal to at least one additional potentially toxic agent.

Obviously the use of procedures that either actually or virtually remove the offending chemical requires that profound emesis has not already occurred and unabsorbed amounts of the offending chemical are believed to be in the stomach. The interval of time between ingestion of the offending chemical and the use of these procedures should be reasonable in order to ensure that the agent is still in the stomach, since that portion of the chemical which has passed into the upper intestine would be beyond immediate reach by the procedure.

There is only a limited amount of clinical evidence to establish the effectiveness under practical conditions for most of the procedures that have been described. A rational approach to the use of these procedures would be that if there is good evidence, on the basis of history and physical examination of the subject, to support the belief that potentially lethal or seriously excessive quantities of an agent had been consumed and that some of the chemical was still in the stomach, one or more of the above procedures should be instituted to terminate further absorption of the offending chemical. This rationale would apply even in the presence of serious necrotic destruction of the esophagus or stomach. In the latter case, it would be more appropriate to avoid emetics. Orally administered chemical adsorbents and neutralizing agents would be preferred, to avoid the additional insult and possible perforation of the necrotized esophagus and stomach produced by gastric lavage.

Direct removal of unabsorbed amounts of a potentially toxic material from the intestinal tract is impractical. When unabsorbed material is present in the intestinal tract, procedures are used that are directed toward the prevention of absorption and the hastening of transport of the chemical through the intestinal tract so that it is eliminated in the excreta. Despite the lack of specific information on the effectiveness of such procedures, there is a rational basis for the use of cathartics and adsorbents in these cases. Poorly absorbable, innocuous materials, such as liquid petrolatum which is a solvent for fat-soluble agents and which also has a low-order cathartic activity, may effectively carry a fat-soluble offending agent through the intestinal tract, thereby limiting its absorption. The more rapid-acting cathartics, such as sodium sulfate or magnesium hydroxide, also function to hasten the transit of intestinal contents. When the insulting chemical is a slowly absorbed agent, such procedures may effectively remove the chemical from the body before absorption can be complete.

In addition to the measures used to prevent translocation of toxicants from the intestinal tract to the blood stream, there are antidotal mechanisms that influence translocation of the chemical from the blood stream to effector sites. An excellent example of such a mechanism is demonstrated in the prevention (and treatment) of cyanide intoxication, whereby the use of antidotal agents is directed toward preventing the cyanide from gaining access to the receptor sites. The brief description of cyanide toxicity which follows will help to clarify the concept that an antidotal agent can be more effective in preventing a toxic effect than in treating the toxic effect of a chemical intoxicant.

Although cyanide reacts with a number of metal-containing enzymes, it owes its toxicity primarily to its ability to react and form a stable complex with the iron in ferric cytochrome oxidase. This enzyme is thereby inhibited. Since aerobic metabolism is dependent on this enzyme system, the tissues can no longer utilize oxygen and the tissues suffer from hypoxia. Protection of the animal from the toxic effect of the cyanide is accomplished by diverting the cyanide before it reacts with the cytochrome enzyme. This diversion is accomplished by promoting the formation of additional sources of ferric iron which will react with cyanide, leading to the formation of less toxic cyanide products. The procedure is to administer nitrite, either as inhaled amyl nitrite or injected sodium nitrite, which causes the formation of methemoglobin by promoting the conversion of the ferrous iron in hemoglobin to ferric iron. The reactions are as follows.

$$\text{Hemoglobin (Fe}^{2+}) \xrightarrow{\text{ nitrite }} \begin{array}{c} \text{Cyanide} \\ + \\ \text{Methemoglobin (Fe}^{3+}) \\ \downarrow \\ \text{Cyanmethemoglobin} \end{array}$$

In addition to the use of nitrite, current therapy of potential cyanide intoxication also involves converting the cyanide to the less toxic thiocyanate. Normally, the body is capable of detoxifying cyanide by converting it to thiocyanate by the action of the liver enzyme rhodanase in the presence of sulfur. In the therapy of cyanide intoxication, the sulfur is made available by administration of sodium thiosulfate and the reaction is as follows.

$$\text{cyanide} + \text{thiosulfate} \rightarrow \text{thiocyanate}$$

Under experimental conditions, dogs can be protected from 20 LD_{50}'s of sodium cyanide by pretreatment with thiosulfate plus nitrite. Thiosulfate plus nitrite therapy effectively alters the translocation and detoxifies the cyanide radical before it can gain access to the receptor sites and thereby effectively decreases the slope of the ascending portion of the toxicity curve shown in Fig. 11.1B.

Whenever biotransformation of a compound results in the formation of a product that is more toxic than the initial compound, blockade or inhibition of the biotransforming system would theoretically reduce the availability of the toxic product. This is an additional system that would favorably influence the slope of the ascending portion of the toxicity curve shown in Fig. 11.1*B*. One example of this is the use of ethanol in the treatment of methanol intoxication. Methanol is prone to produce blindness in humans and other primates. The blindness is due to destruction of the retina and degeneration of the optic nerve. It appears that a metabolite of methanol and not the unchanged methanol is responsible for the blindness. It is also clear that in humans and other primates both ethanol and methanol are primarily oxidized by the same enzyme, namely alcohol dehydrogenase (ADH). ADH is localized most abundantly in the liver and it converts ethanol to acetaldehyde and methanol to formaldehyde with subsequent conversion of the formaldehyde to formic acid. The acidosis created by the presence of formic acid is a major problem, in addition to the blindness involved in the toxicity from ingestion of methanol. Ethanol is the preferred substrate for the enzyme ADH and is metabolized several times more rapidly than is methanol. When both alcohols are present at the same time, they compete for the enzyme and in this manner the rate of metabolism of methanol is suppressed so that the concentration of toxic metabolites is also diminished. Ethanol must be used with caution in any patient severely affected with methanol because both agents are depressant drugs and their depressant effects will summate in direct relation to the concentrations of the agents that are present.

PROCEDURES FOR ENHANCING TERMINATION OF ACTION OR ELIMINATION

In inhalation toxicology, the management of carbon monoxide intoxication in humans is an example of the principle of enhancing the termination of action of an agent as a means of treatment of the intoxication. Carbon monoxide produces toxicity when it is inhaled by virtue of its ability to compete with oxygen in binding with hemoglobin and certain respiratory enzymes, thereby resulting in a diminished availability of oxygen in the tissues. Since the combination of carbon monoxide with hemoglobin and the respiratory enzymes is readily reversible in the presence of an adequate amount of oxygen, treatment of carbon monoxide intoxication involves administration of oxygen. The affinity of oxygen for the hemoglobin receptor site is about 200 times less than the affinity of the same site for carbon monoxide. Therefore, the effectiveness of oxygen therapy is a function of the concentration of oxygen that is used as the antidotal procedure. The time required to remove half of the carbon monoxide from the blood is about 300 min when the person is allowed to breathe atmospheric air (containing 20% oxygen) that is free of carbon monoxide, whereas by administration of pure oxygen it only takes approximately 80 min to eliminate half of the carbon monoxide from the blood; under hyperbaric conditions of three atmospheres of pure oxygen, 50% of the carbon monoxide will be cleared in 25 min. This same principle applies for any antidotal agent that acts by competitively displacing a toxicant from its receptor so that, in effect, the rate of elimination of the toxicant is increased.

Absorption of a toxic quantity of an agent from the gastrointestinal tract or from topical sites of administration and some degree of equilibrium with the various tissues in the animal occur concomitantly, resulting in the appearance of the subjective and objective harmful effects characteristic of that chemical. Antidotal procedures at this level of intoxication may consist of actual and virtual removal of the offending chemical from the effector sites. If the reaction between the chemical and the effector substance is a reversible one, removal of the chemical can be accomplished by lowering the concentration of the chemical in the extracellular compartments of the animal. Under these conditions actual removal is achieved by enhancement of excretion of the compound from the body.

Since the kidney is the predominant route of excretion of foreign chemicals or their metabolites (except gases, for which the lungs are the primary route of excretion), effective enhancement of excretion of chemicals by the kidneys is accomplished according to mechanisms outlined in Chapter 3. The kidney functions to form urine by the combined processes of ultrafiltration of the blood, active and passive reabsorption of the filtrate, and secretion from the blood to the filtrate. Many foreign chemicals are readily filtered and are reabsorbed by the blood from the filtrate.

The procedure of increasing urine formation by the induction of water diureses enhances the rate of excretion of many foreign compounds only to a minor degree. Diuresis produced by osmotic diuretics, such as urea or mannitol, is somewhat more effective. Urinary excretion of an organic electrolyte, however, can be significantly enhanced by adjusting the pH of the urine to favor ionization of the compound. Therefore, excretion in the urine of a weak organic acid, such as acetylsalicylic acid ($pK_a = 3.5$), is enhanced if the urine is alkalinized (see Fig. 4.1), and excretion of a weak organic base, such as quinine ($pK_a = 8.4$), is enhanced if the urine is acidified. If the pK_a of a compound is known, and provided the undissociated part of the substance is to some extent lipid-soluble, it is possible to predict the effect of altering the urinary pH on the excretion of the compound through calculations as described in Chapter 4. The effectiveness of this technique has been well established for salicylate and barbiturate intoxication.

In addition to removal of a chemical from the circulation by enhancement of excretion by the kidney, many chemicals can be removed by the use of chemical–mechanical dialyzing devices, which substitute for or supplement the function of the kidney. Examples are the artificial kidney or peritoneal dialysis equipment. In acute, severe barbiturate intoxication, the artificial kidney is an effective device for the removal of barbiturate from the blood. Because of the limited availability of artificial kidneys, this procedure has limited emergency use. Peritoneal hemodialysis, a much simpler procedure, basically involves irrigating the peritoneal cavity with a dialyzing fluid.

Hemoperfusion is a direct method of lowering the blood concentration of several xenobiotic agents when they are the cause of intoxication. This procedure uses cartridges containing activated charcoal. Arterial blood from a patient is introduced directly into the cartridge so that it comes in contact with the charcoal. Xenobiotics as well as many of their biotransformation products may be absorbed on the charcoal, depending on their affinity for the charcoal. The blood then flows back into the patient's venous circulation. Arterial pressure maintains a continuous flow of blood through the cartridge, resulting in a gradual decrease in the body load of the intoxicant. This procedure has only a limited use in the clinic, but it has been used in the treatment of barbiturate and carbamazepine intoxication. Complications that occur are associated with concomitant removal of blood cells (lymphocytes and thrombocytes) from the blood by the charcoal.

Since many chemicals of toxicologic interest have specific sites of action which are responsible for toxicity of the chemical in the biologic specimen, removal of the chemical from specific sites of action terminates the undesirable effect of the chemical. Removal of the chemical from other binding sites (nonspecific), together with detoxication of the compound by combining it with antidote, inactivates the compound in the animal. It is not necessary to enhance excretion of the chemical from the animal to effectively terminate the action of the compound at the effector site. This type of antidotal therapy, the most effective known, involves the use of antidotal chemicals that directly or indirectly produce less toxic complexes with the offending agent. Examples of such antidotal agents are "British Antilewisite" (BAL, or dimercaprol) and EDTA for the treatment of heavy metal intoxication, and the oximes for the treatment of organic phosphate intoxication.

The heavy metals most commonly encountered in clinical toxicology are mercury, lead, and arsenic. These metals owe their toxicity primarily to their ability to react with and inhibit sulfhydryl enzyme systems involved in several vital processes in the body, such as those involved in the production of cellular energy. Antidotal therapy of such intoxications is based on either the administration of simple dithiol compounds as exemplified by BAL, or chelation as exemplified by EDTA. BAL and EDTA are capable of forming metal complexes more stable than the enzyme–metal complex. In the case of the arsenic enzyme complex, the product is a monothiol complex whereas the dithiol, BAL, causes the formation of a cyclic thioarsenate according to the following reaction.

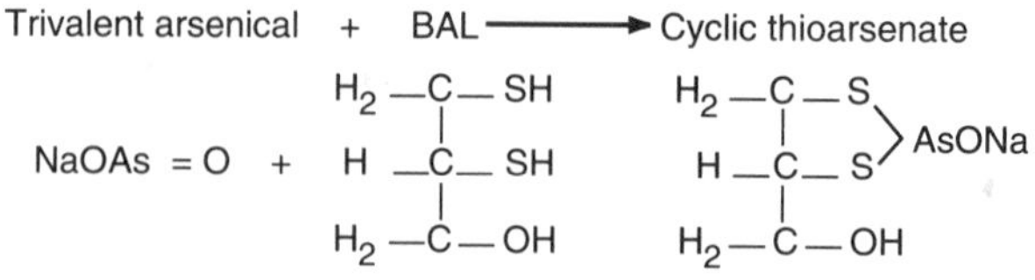

Trivalent arsenical   +   BAL ⟶ Cyclic thioarsenate

$$
NaOAs = O \; + \;
\begin{array}{l}
H_2 - C - SH \\
\;\;\;\;\; | \\
H - C - SH \\
\;\;\;\;\; | \\
H_2 - C - OH
\end{array}
\qquad
\begin{array}{l}
H_2 - C - S \\
\;\;\;\;\; | \quad \;\; \rangle AsONa \\
H - C - S \\
\;\;\;\;\; | \\
H_2 - C - OH
\end{array}
$$

In the case of lead intoxication, the use of the calcium chelate of disodium EDTA acts as an ion exchanger in which the calcium is exchanged for the heavy metal ion and a soluble and stable chelate of lead is formed. As a chelate, lead is nonionized, and this chelate is available for excretion by the kidney as a ring complex. This reaction is shown below.

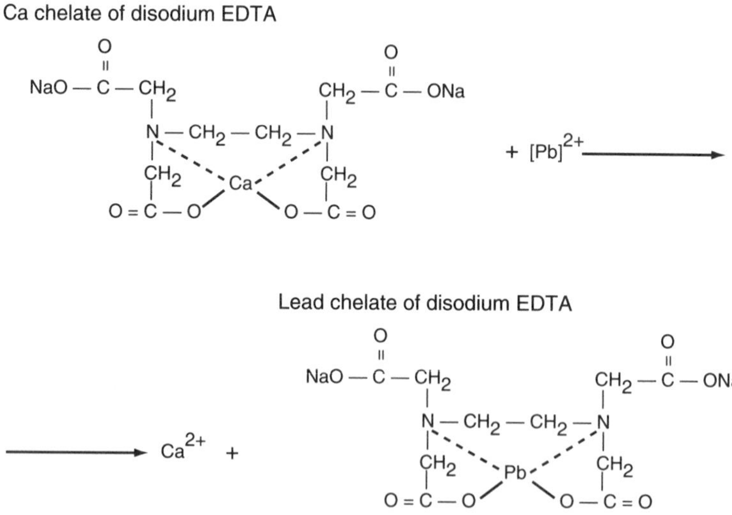

Ca chelate of disodium EDTA

+ [Pb]$^{2+}$ ⟶

Lead chelate of disodium EDTA

⟶ Ca^{2+} +

In both examples, the combined form of the metal encompasses an unionized form of the metal. This complex is stable and is a less toxic molecule. Following the administration of EDTA, the rate of excretion of lead as the EDTA complex in the urine of patients intoxicated with lead may increase as much as 50-fold above the normal untreated excretion rate. Therefore, chelation therapy not only serves to detoxify the lead and withdraw it from the effector sites, but also promotes elimination of the metal from the animal.

One of the most significant developments in antidotal therapy is the adoption of nucleophilic compounds in the treatment of organic phosphate intoxication. Early work in this field indicated that hydroxamic acids would displace phosphorus from the phosphorylated cholinesterase by reacting with the complexed enzyme, and the product would undergo hydrolysis resulting in release of the active enzyme. In 1955 reports appeared demonstrating the high order of effectiveness of pyridine-2-aldoxime methiodide as such a nucleophilic-reactivating agent for phosphorylated cholinesterase.

Several organic phosphate agents are used extensively as pesticides. These agents owe their high order of toxicity in intact biologic specimens to the fact that they readily react with and inactivate enzymes of the cholinesterase type by phosphorylating the enzyme. These enzymes, and particularly acetylcholinesterase, are important in regard to maintenance of impulse transfer between nerve cells as well as between nerve and skeletal muscle cells in most, if not all, species of biologic specimens that have nerve systems. Acetylcholinesterase functions to terminate the action of the neurohumor (acetylcholine) which is liberated at the end of the nerve. When acetylcholinesterase is inhibited by an organic phosphate, the neurohumor (acetylcholine) is believed to accumulate at the nerve ending so that transfer of nerve impulses across synapses at the autonomic ganglia and at the nerve-muscle junctions is prevented.

The sequence of reactions leading to phosphorylation and thus inactivation of cholinesterase by the organic phosphate diisopropylfluorophosphate (DFP), and the reaction involved in regeneration of the phosphorylated enzyme by the use of the oxime pyridine-2-aldoxime methiodide (2-PAM) are shown in Fig. 11.2. In the figure, the enzyme is depicted as having two active sites, one of which is the anionic site and the other an esteratic site. Reaction 1 leads to the formation of the phosphorylated (inhibited) enzyme in which the phosphate is attached to the esteratic site of the enzyme. When the inhibited enzyme reacts with the oxime (Reaction 2), the unoccupied anionic site on the enzyme serves to orient the oxime so that it combines with the phosphorus to form a product that undergoes hydrolysis (Reaction 3), resulting in liberation of a regenerated active enzyme. The oxime therefore functions as an antidotal agent by displacing the phosphorus from the enzyme. In the absence of additional organic phosphate, which could in turn rephosphorylate the enzyme, oxime therapy will return the cholinesterase-dependent physiological mechanism to normal.

The use of biologic antibodies (antitoxins) as antidotal agents is an important area in antidotal therapy but it has been generally applicable only in cases involving bacterial toxins. However, in the mid 1970s an

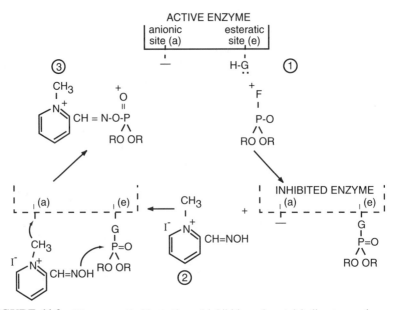

FIGURE 11.2   Diagrammatic illustration of inhibition of acetylcholinesterase (enzyme) with diisopropylfluorophosphate (Reaction 1) and reaction of the phosphorylated enzyme with 2-pyridine aldoxime methiodide (Reaction 2) and hydrolysis of the product of Reaction 2 which results in regeneration of active enzyme (Reaction 3). (Adapted from concepts of Wilson, I. B., *J. Am. Chem. Soc.* **77**:2385, 1955; and Jandorf, B. J., *J. Am. Chem. Soc.* **78**:3686, 1956.)

antibody fragment was prepared and successfully used in the treatment of digoxin intoxication. The antibody to digoxin was prepared by immunizing sheep with a digoxin–serum albumin conjugate. The immune globulin that was produced in the blood of the sheep was cleaved into fragments, one of which was found to have a high affinity for digoxin. The digoxin–antibody complex is excreted in the urine, thereby lowering the body load of digoxin. Currently it is the recommended antidote for digoxin intoxication. It is commonly known as the Fab antibody, that is, the Fragment a b antibody.

PROCEDURES FOR ELEVATING THE THRESHOLD OF TOXICITY

According to Fig. 11.1D, elevation of the threshold of toxicity without changing the concentration of the chemical at the effector site would abolish the toxicity of an offending chemical. Elevation of the threshold of toxicity is practically achieved with antidotal chemicals in two ways. One is to directly antagonize the system affected by the toxicity through enhancement of a physiologically opposing system. The other method is to use one of several drugs known to actually block the response produced by the presence of other drugs by an action on the same physiological mechanism. These mechanisms are clarified in the following paragraphs by use of examples.

The presence of physiologically antagonistic systems is common in most animals. Antagonistic muscle systems enable movement of structures and antagonistic nerve systems enable excitation or inhibition of organ systems. Drugs have been designed with the specific objective of having an effect on one or more of such antagonistic systems. The proper use of drugs that affect opposing physiological mechanisms for antidotal therapeutic purposes involves an extensive understanding of pharmacology. These drugs have known mechanisms of action and usually, when used as antidotes, they are used for the purpose of controlling harmful symptoms.

Generally the use of drugs that affect antagonistic physiological mechanisms is of greater academic interest than it is of practical value. This is probably because it is technically difficult to titrate a drug effect on one system against an existing effect of a chemical on an opposing system. Therefore, although there is considerable evidence that under highly controlled laboratory conditions, severe respiratory depression induced by barbiturates can be effectively antagonized by drugs such as picrotoxin or pentylene tetrazol, it has been demonstrated that under clinical conditions respiratory depression is more efficiently controlled by mechanical support of respiration.

In contrast to this, a simple fall in blood pressure that occurs following severe barbiturate intoxication can be effectively antagonized by intravenous administration of norepinephrine, both in the laboratory and in the clinic. Each of these examples involves the use of a drug that stimulates a physiological mechanism that is antagonistic to the system affected by the offending chemical. In each case, the offending chemical continues to exert its effect at its site of action, but the effect is overcome by the effect of the antidotal agent on an opposing physiological system.

In contrast to the pharmacologic antagonists that act on opposing physiological mechanisms, there are many drugs whose pharmacologic effect can be specifically blocked by an action of a second drug on the same mechanism. Insofar as antidotal concepts are concerned, the basis for drug action is that drugs that affect physiological mechanisms produce their effects by combining with "receptors." The drug–receptor combination either directly induces a response or initiates the formation of a product which causes a response. These reactions are analogous to conventional enzyme substrate reactions as follows.

(1) Drug + Receptor⟶ Drug — Receptor Complex⟶ Product⟶ Response
(2) Enzyme + Substrate ⟶ Enzyme — Substrate Complex ⟶ Product

Obviously the drug (or foreign chemical) action can be prevented if the drug is displaced from the receptor or if the same chemical sites on the receptor are occupied by an antidotal substance that does not initiate a physiological response.

An example of the competitive type of antidotal therapy is the use of naloxone as an antidote to the effects of morphine on respiration. In this case, morphine reacts with the receptor (respiratory center in the brain) and the product of this reaction produces the respiratory depression. Theoretically naloxone also reacts with and displaces morphine from the same receptor, but the product of this reaction has considerably less respiratory depressant effect. By a similar mechanism, morphine-induced narcosis can be reversed by the antidote and withdrawal symptoms can be induced in morphine addicts by the administration of naloxone.

Another example of displacement of one drug from a receptor by another is the use of vitamin K as an antagonist to the toxic effect of the anticoagulant drug Dicumarol. The receptor for Dicumarol in this instance is an unidentified enzyme system, which is present in the liver and for which vitamin K is the normal substrate. Vitamin K plus the enzyme yields an enzyme–substrate complex that is normally essential for the production of certain proteins, such as prothrombin and convertin, which are necessary for the normal coagulation of the blood. Dicumarol reacts with the same enzyme system, but this reaction fails to produce the proteins necessary for the coagulation of blood. Therefore, excessive doses of Dicumarol would create a tendency to hemorrhage from only minor injuries, or would even cause spontaneous hemorrhage.

A sufficient amount of vitamin K is an effective antidote to Dicumarol-induced hemorrhage, since it will compete with and displace Dicumarol from the enzyme complex and reestablish normal formation of the coagulation factors of the blood. Thus, vitamin K and Dicumarol appear to be mutually antagonistic on the receptor (enzyme) mechanism on the basis of a displacement by mass action and affinity for the enzyme system. In pharmacology, such antagonistic chemicals are referred to as competitive antagonists on an enzyme system.

In the foregoing two examples, the offending chemical is not detoxified. Rather, the concentration representing the threshold at which they are capable of producing a harmful effect is elevated by the presence of the antidotal agent.

An additional example of the use of the antidotal chemicals to elevate the threshold of toxicity is the use of atropine as an antidote to certain responses in intoxication with muscarine, which is partially responsible for one type of mushroom (*Aminata muscaria*) poisoning. One theory of the mechanism of induction of toxicity from the alkaloid muscarine is that muscarine reacts with the same receptor through which acetylcholine induces its effect. The muscarine–receptor complex initiates physiological responses that are similar to those induced by acetylcholine at the autonomic nerve endings, such as slowing of the heart, decrease in blood pressure, excessive salivation, and constriction of the airway in the lungs.

These effects of muscarine can be prevented by the administration of atropine which combines with the same receptor. Atropine either displaces the muscarine from the receptor or prevents the muscarine–receptor complex from producing a product that is in turn responsible for the physiological effects. Atropine does not directly react with, inactivate, or detoxify the muscarine molecule. Rather, the concentration of muscarine necessary to reach the threshold at which the toxic response occurs is greatly elevated by the presence of atropine. This concept is supported by experimental evidence obtained under laboratory conditions, which indicates that the pharmacologic effects of muscarine can be titrated against those of atropine.

A popular misconception is that concerned with the general use of chemical agents for specific antidotal therapy. There is no single agent or combination of agents that can be used as a universally effective chemical antidote. Some of the specific antidotal chemicals have been discussed in the foregoing examples. Such agents are used only when a diagnosis can be made in which the agent responsible for the toxicity can be absolutely identified. Even then, only in a relatively few cases is the toxicant one for which a specific antidotal agent is available for immediate use except in a few emergency clinics. In many cases of chemical intoxication in humans the causative toxicant can only be suspected on the basis of a history of possible exposure and the presence of certain symptoms. Of all cases of chemical intoxication encountered clinically, specific chemical antidotal therapy is possible for only relatively few.

No specific antidotal agents are known for the large majority of the commonly encountered harmful chemicals. In the absence of specific antidotal agents or definite knowledge of the nature of the chemical involved in a specific case, treatment of chemical intoxication is primarily directed toward limiting absorption of the chemical by either removing the chemical from the subject or removing the subject from the exposure to the chemical (as in the case of contaminated environments) and by supporting the vital functions of the body (such as blood pressure and respiration) as needed so that as time passes, normal detoxication and excretion mechanisms terminate the presence of the offending chemical in the body. Furthermore, even under those conditions for which specific antidotal chemicals are known, improperly used antidotes are also capable of producing harmful effects. Therefore, employment of physiologically active antidotes is subject to their knowledgeable use, so that the objectives of therapy are achieved without induction of added chemical injury. The use of antidotal chemicals is therefore restricted to those cases in which irreparable damage or death is imminent and in which normal detoxication and excretion mechanisms are unable to cope with the excessive quantities of the harmful chemical.

CHAPTER **12**

Principles of Biological Tests for Toxicity

GENERAL PRINCIPLES

Toxicology has been defined as the study of the effects of chemical agents on biological material with special emphasis on harmful effects. It basically involves an understanding of all effects of essentially all chemicals on all types of living matter. There is ample evidence to indicate that every chemical is capable, under some conditions, of producing some type of effect on every biological tissue. Toxicologic tests are therefore the tests that define the conditions that must be present when a biological cell is affected by a given chemical entity, and the nature of the effect which is produced. As far as the conditions that must be present are concerned, they may vary from being practically unattainable in ordinary circumstances to being so readily attained that simple exposure of living tissue to certain chemicals produces destruction of the cells. As far as the nature of any effect of a chemical on living tissue is concerned, effects may be of such minor significance that the tissue is able to carry on its ordinary function in a normal manner so that it is only under conditions of stress or critical tests that a chemical-induced effect is even detectable. Effects may result from small amounts of some chemicals whereas large amounts of other compounds may be required to produce any positive untoward finding. Generally it is a simple matter to separate those relatively few chemicals that in small amounts produce prompt effects that are distinctly harmful to living cells from those that are practically harmless when exposure is over a short period of time, but it becomes difficult to demonstrate that small amounts of some compounds do not produce some types of toxicity when animals are exposed over a long period of time.

Most of the biological methods which have been developed in toxicology are the result of the practical need to obtain as much information as possible about the effects of chemicals insofar as they may be pertinent to man's continued physical well-being. The continuing economic progress of the human race has been accompanied by a continuing increase in the numbers of chemical entities to which man is either intentionally or unintentionally exposed. A person may be exposed through direct industrial or domestic occupational contact, through contact with the clothes or devices he wears, the food, liquid, and drugs he consumes, and the atmosphere he inhales. It is necessary not only to understand the toxicities that can occur but also to obtain assurance that exposure of man to large numbers of chemical entities will not lead to obvious direct or insidious indirect detrimental effects. Consequently it is essential that some toxicity data be acquired on all chemical agents. For those chemicals which are to be intentionally administered to man, such as food additives, food substitutes, or drugs, it is necessary to obtain as many toxicity data as is economically possible.

Because of the moral, ethical, and legal restrictions regarding the use of humans for experimental purposes in order to acquire toxicologic data, only limited amounts of such data are available. Information regarding the effects of chemicals on humans is obtainable only after a chemical is used by humans or from limited types of experimental procedures that may be conducted on humans. Biological methods in toxicology therefore generally involve the use of expendable species of animals on the hypothesis that toxicity studies in suitable species have an extrapolative value for man.

Several of the procedures involved in testing for toxicity involve the use of nonmammalian species and even cell cultures. It would be of great advantage to be able to utilize such species as bacteria, neurospora, daphnia, drosophila, the various echinoderms, or fish for evaluation of toxicity because of the economic advantage and abundance of such populations of living cells. Furthermore, some of these species lend themselves to accurate and simple procedures such as those that make use of their accurately defined and measurable genetic characteristics, reproductive processes, and enzymatic performance. The main drawbacks associated with the use of such species are the dissimilarities in translocation barriers as compared to man and differences in or the lack of biotransformation mechanisms that are present in man. These factors preclude extrapolation of the data obtained on most nonmammalian species to man. Nevertheless such tests serve the purpose of alerting the investigator to potential toxic hazards which then can be further studied in mammalian species. When any chemical is used in massive quantities such as in agriculture and becomes available in the general environment, it is necessary to evaluate the toxicity of that agent in many species which may directly or indirectly influence the overall welfare of man.

It should be recognized that there are many variations in both short- and long-term chemical-induced toxicity among various mammalian species of animals; however, careful and complete evaluation of the effects of chemicals on animals has been shown to be the most rational, acceptable, and successful means of determining most types of toxicity for purposes of extrapolation to man.

PRINCIPLES OF EXPERIMENTAL TOXICOLOGIC METHODOLOGY

The principles of toxicologic methodology are based on the premise that all effects of chemicals on living tissues are the result of a reaction with or interaction between any given chemical entity and some component of the living biologic system. This initial reaction may not be evident. The result of this reaction is manifested as an effect on the function, and in many cases the structure, of the biologic system. The effect on function may not necessarily be accompanied by a detectable change in structure of the biologic system, that is, it may be only a biochemical lesion. The effect may be reversible in the absence of continued exposure to the chemical or it may result in death of the cell. The study of toxicological methods is centered on the detection and evaluation of the nature of the chemical-induced changes in function and structure and the significance of these effects on living cells. Since all effects of chemicals on living systems are not necessarily harmful effects, a principal function of the science of toxicology is to identify clearly those chemicals capable of producing serious harm to living systems. As a science, toxicology has developed a methodology to detect chemical-induced alterations in function and structure of living systems, to investigate many of the factors that determine how chemicals gain access to biological cells, to establish the parameters of the conditions under which various chemicals do or do not produce biologic effects, and to define the mechanisms by which chemicals interact with the various components of living systems in order to directly or indirectly produce toxic effects.

As a result of the development of this toxicologic methodology, certain general principles have become apparent. These principles apply to many, and perhaps all, toxicologic test procedures. They are as follows:

1. In order for a chemical to produce a biologic effect, it must come into immediate contact with the biological cells (or receptors) under consideration.

2. For each chemical there exists a quantity below which it produces no detectable effect on all biologic systems, and a quantity at which it produces a significant effect on all biologic systems. Between these extremes lies the range of quantities at which each chemical will exert a significant effect on some types of biologic systems.

3. Cells having similar functions and similar metabolic pathways in various species generally will be affected similarly by a given chemical entity.

4. Small changes in the structure of a chemical agent may greatly influence the biological action of that agent.

These principles have been introduced in previous chapters and will be considered here only in regard to how they contribute to an understanding of the various test procedures that are used in toxicology.

TRANSLOCATION FACTORS IN TOXICOLOGIC TESTS

The discussion in Chapter 3 has defined the main factors that are involved in the transfer of a chemical to various compartments within an animal. The principle which states that chemicals must come in contact with the biologic system in order to have an effect on the system would be a simple and obvious one if all biologic systems consisted only of a solution of living material in some universal solvent. Such is not the case, since even the simplest single living cell consists of both suspended and dissolved material in a highly selective solvent, all of which are encased in a membrane. The total complex is characterized by its ability to carry on a series of functions that make it a "living cell." In progressing from the single-celled organism to the multicelled organism and on to the many tissue and multiorgan type of biologic specimen, particles within cells become encased in membranes so the membranes increase in number, cells become encased in organs and the organs encased in other tissue so that the final biologic form becomes a protected unit that lives within its own internal and usually closely regulated environment. In order for a foreign chemical to exert an effect other than at its site of application, it must gain access to the various parts of this internal environment. Therefore it must necessarily be translocated to the various parts of the animal, tissue, or cell.

In a complex biologic system such as man, those chemicals which are absorbed neither through the skin nor from the gastrointestinal tract would be innocuous if applied to the skin or consumed by mouth except for whatever action they may exert on the skin or in the gastrointestinal lining. In contrast to this, if such a chemical were injected through the skin or into the bloodstream, or inhaled into the lungs, and if it were translocated to all cells in the internal environment, it could potentially exert an effect at essentially any site within the body. In the case of those chemical agents that are used as drugs for therapeutic purposes, the biologic barriers to translocation of the agent may be so effective that in order to get a therapeutic effect from the drug, it must be administered by injection methods. Therefore, the methods used for a reasonably complete evaluation of the toxicity of any chemical agent necessarily involve administering the agent to the experimental animal by a variety of routes. The route by which the agent would be expected to come in contact with the biologic specimen under the conditions of practical use of the chemical would necessarily be included in the test procedure. That is, experimental programs using animals involving the route of intended use of any chemical would be expected to provide the most acceptable data for practical extrapolative use to man if the compound is intended for use by man. When new chemical entities are not intended for use by humans, the experiments of greatest practical value are those that simulate the routes by which accidental exposure to the chemical could occur if the intention of the experiments is to obtain data to evaluate toxicity or ensure safety to man.

Certain compounds commonly are referred to as being biologically inert, but such compounds are inert only in the sense that under ordinary conditions they do not gain access to the cells. Usually this is because they are insoluble in biological fluids. In such cases, these chemicals, if present in sufficient concentration, still could affect cells in a mechanical traumatic manner. Examples of such agents are the metals, natural minerals, and highly nonreactive plastic polymers. However, agents which are insoluble in the biological fluids, if implanted in a biologic specimen, will elicit some response in the cells even if it is no more than a response to a "foreign" body. The principle under consideration is intended to be valid only under the condition that the chemical entity is soluble to some degree in biological fluids. Its action on cells may be basically nonspecific, that is, changing the total ion strength or pH, or simply occupying space. Obviously, in a multicelled organism, any effect of a chemical on one type of cell may indirectly influence other cells in the organism since the organism must maintain all cells in a viable and normally functioning state if absolute, total, normal function is to be maintained.

The chemical agents that are of significant toxicologic interest are usually compounds which are soluble in the fluid phases of biologic systems and are therefore potentially available to the cells. The solubility of such compounds in body water may be very small. Although in all biologic systems the fluid phase is mainly water, the systems also contain protein and lipid or lipid-like material as well as a number of inorganic ions. The protein may loosely bind to the chemical and the lipid may serve as a significant solvent for the transport of the chemical agent involved. In fact, most drugs are weak organic acids or bases, and as such are frequently soluble in lipids. Furthermore, in many animals such lipid-soluble agents frequently are biotransformed by oxidative enzyme systems to water-soluble derivatives which may have either more or less toxic potential than the parent compound. The study of the toxicity of any chemical entity is necessarily a study of any products which may arise as a result of changes (biotransformation) in the chemical which are induced by the test animal. In this manner, although some degree of solubility of any chemical agent in body fluids is essential if it is to be translocated, the compound does not necessarily have to be soluble in water. Such agents may be carried on protein, dissolved in lipids, or biotransformed to different derivatives which have different solubility characteristics. The general principle under consideration stipulates that under some conditions all cells will be affected by chemicals which come in contact with them. The effect which is manifested may be different in different cells, just as the concentration of the compound which is necessary to produce an effect may be different in different types of cells.

CONCENTRATION–RESPONSE FACTORS IN TOXICOLOGIC TESTS

The second general principle is concerned with the fact that there is some minimal amount of each chemical agent below which there is no effect on biologic systems and that there is a greater amount of each chemical at which a significant effect will be present on essentially all living systems.

Whenever the effect of a chemical is determined on a single experimental animal, two types of data may be obtained. One of these is the all-or-none type of data in which an effect is either present or absent (e.g., the animal either lives or dies). The second type of data is the graded response type in which an effect is present but may be of a specific intensity, such as impairment of some type of performance, decrease in heart rate, or even an increase in the number of tumors. The latter type of effects must always be quantitated. This is frequently done for any given effect in terms of percentage of normal or in terms of incidence of occurrence in a given group of test animals. The more sophisticated the experiment the more the graded effect may be quantitated. In either type of experimental data, the information is quantitative in nature.

Toxicologic experiments are generally not conducted on a single animal. Whenever an experiment is conducted, it usually involves the use of a selected number of experimental animals (or biologic preparations) rather than a single animal. Also, the quantity of the chemical agent under consideration which is administered to the animals will be varied in different groups of the animals. Therefore, all experimental toxicologic data are obtained by administering a series of progressively increasing amounts of a chemical to different groups in which each group contains specific numbers of experimental biological preparations or whole animals. When this is done under actual laboratory conditions and data regarding effects of the chemical are obtained, the data consist of measurable responses in each group from each selected quantity of the chemical. Regardless of the chemical under consideration, if an all-or-none type of response, such as lethality, is one datum which is obtained, there will be some minimal quantity below which none of the animals in the group will die. At some intermediate quantity, a portion of the group of animals receiving that dose will die, but not all of them will die. Therefore, although this latter quantity produces an all-or-none response, in each test the data represent a graded response when groups of animals compose the test population. This variation in response between biologic test specimens within a given species is well established. It is generally referred to as "biological variation" and is to be recognized as being different from "species variation" in response to chemicals.

Toxicologists are accustomed to administering chemicals to experimental animals in specific quantities at specific intervals of time, and the quantity is referred to as the "dose" of the chemical. The terminology used to identify doses varies with the type of chemical. If the chemical is a solid, it is administered to the test animals in terms of weight, or it may be dissolved in a solvent such as water whereby the quantity is then defined as given volume of a known concentration of the chemical in solution. If it is a liquid, it may be in terms of weight or volume of the chemical. If it is a gas, it is usually in terms of volume or concentration of the gas in a mixture of gases, such as air. Furthermore, the quantity is further defined in terms of quantity per unit weight or per unit of body surface area of the test animal. Occasionally the interval of time over which the dose is administered is necessarily part of the dose terminology. Conventional examples of doses are grams or milligrams per kilogram of body weight or per square meter of body surface area, milliliters or cubic centimeters of a solution per kilogram of body weight or per square meter of body surface area, or parts per million (ppm) or millimoles per liter of a gas in air or other gases.

When comparative dose–response relations are made between species of animals and man, there is some evidence that the best correlation is obtained by comparing doses on the basis of body surface area rather than on the basis of animal weight. Table 12.1 compares some of the more common experimental laboratory animals with man in regard to the effect of their relative weights and body surface areas on the dose of certain chemical agents of toxicologic interest.

If there were no biological barriers or other factors which would affect the equal distribution of a chemical throughout a biological specimen, then the quantity of the chemical represented by the dose would be related directly to the concentration of the chemical in most compartments of the specimen. Although this is true for some chemicals it is more frequently not true for the majority of chemicals, particularly when the test specimen consists of a whole animal. The factors that influence distribution of a dose of a chemical in the animal are:

1. Membranous barriers to translocation.
2. Selective storage depots such as binding to proteins or selective partitioning into lipids.
3. Concentration-dependent metabolic inactivation.
4. Excretion.

These factors are responsible for a continuous variation in the distribution of a chemical in the various compartments of an animal so that at any given time there may be great differences in concentration of the chemical

TABLE 12.1 Relative Sensitivity of Man as Compared to Some Common Laboratory Animals[a]

Dose on the basis of body weight (mg/kg)		Dose on the basis of body surface area (mg/m²)
MTD in man = $1/12$ LD_{10}	or	$3/4$ LD_{10} mice
MTD in man = $1/9$ LD_{10}	or	$5/7$ LD_{10} in hamsters
MTD in man = $1/7$ LD_{10}	or	$6/7$ LD_{10} in rats
MTD in man = $1/3$ MTD	or	1 MTD in rhesus monkeys
MTD in man = $1/2$ MTD	or	1 MTD in dogs

Note. Toxic dose levels of anticancer drugs when the dose is calculated according to body weight or according to body surface area. Data compiled from retrospective studies reported by Pinkel *et al., Clin. Pharmacol. Ther.* **11**:33, 1970, and from Paget, G. E., *Clinical Testing of New Drugs,* Herrick and Cattell, Eds., p. 33, Revere Publishing Company, New York, 1965. MTD, maximum tolerated dose. LD_{10}, lethal dose for 10% of the animals.

between the various body organs and compartments. However, when a chemical is administered to several members of the same species, the various listed factors may be assumed to be similarly operative in each member of the group. Therefore, if the same dose is administered to more than one member of a single species of animals, that dose may be assumed to distribute itself similarly throughout each compartment within each member of the species. (Unequal distribution between the compartments of two apparently identical members of the same species is probably the principal mechanism which is involved in the phenomenon of biological variation.) The result is that although any biologic effect that is induced by a chemical is related directly to the concentration of the chemical at the site where it can produce its effect, in a given species the concentration is related directly to the dose and therefore there will be a direct relation between dose and effect.

Common usage involves correlation of the effects of chemicals in terms of dose rather than in terms of concentration of the chemical in the animal. In many animal toxicologic studies, the concentration of the chemical at the site where it produces its effect is not known. Therefore, conventional data consist of dose versus effect types of data, that is, dose is plotted versus intensity or incidence of response in the same manner that a concentration–response curve is derived.

At this point it is important to point out that there are some examples of chemical agents that represent exceptions to the concept which has been stated as follows: "It can be readily demonstrated that there is a direct relationship between the frequency of occurrence or intensity of any measurable effect of the chemical on the biological system and the dose or concentration of the chemical agent which is present." The exceptions are uniformly those chemicals that are normally present in the animal. Since the internal environment of all living cells is a rather specific chemical environment involving the presence of specific concentrations of ions and nutrients essential to the life processes of the cells, it follows that depletion of the cells of these substances will lead to harmful consequences or toxicity to the cells. It also follows that there will be a direct relationship between the concentration of the chemical present and the harmful effect on the cell only when the concentration of the chemical is greater than that normally present in the cell. As an example, sufficient depletion of potassium in an animal will produce cardiac arrest and death of the animal and elevation of the depleted potassium concentration to normal will abolish the effect on the heart and prevent death. In contrast to this, if the concentration of potassium is sufficiently elevated above normal, cardiac arrest and consequently death of the animal will occur. In fact, some of the metals that are essential for normal function of animals become known primarily for their toxicity. A good example is selenium which occurs in abundance in the environment and is a cause of illness in animals that eat forage contaminated with salts of this metal. The point to be made is that the response to endogenous chemicals is related directly to the concentration of the chemicals when the concentrations are above normal and indirectly related to the concentrations of the chemicals when the concentrations are below the normal concentration present in the healthy animals. Thus the principle as initially stated is intended to apply to all exogenous (foreign) compounds and to endogenous compounds only when the concentration is greater than normal. As analytical capabilities improve and pharmacodynamics of chemicals and biological systems are better understood, concentration versus effect types of data will become more prevalent, particularly as mechanistic studies are initiated as part of, or complementary to, classical testing protocols.

The dose–response relationship is plotted conventionally by statistical methods as dose of the chemical versus the incidence of occurrence or intensity of an effect. Separate plots are made for experimental data obtained on different species or strains within a species. Figure 12.1 is an example of a log dose–probability plot such as that which would be obtained when lethality of a compound is obtained experimentally following administration of various doses of a chemical to a series of groups of mice. The significance of the slopes of concentration–response relationships is considered elsewhere (see Chapter 2). Regardless of the biological function which is measurably influenced by the chemical, under the practical conditions of an experiment, the proximate intersect of the concentration–response curve of the abscissa (concentration) does not establish the absolute absence of the effect. Obviously the number of animals involved in the test and the degree of experimental perfection in detecting a biologic effect will determine the confidence of the test and therefore the statistical point of intersection of the dose–response curve with the abscissa. However, since the plot is derived statistically, the intersect with the abscissa is a virtual intersect obtained by extrapolation to a proximate zero-effect.

The experimental estimation of the zero-effect or no-effect dose (more properly stated as the no-apparent-effect dose) is the information needed for estimation of the order of safety of any compound under investigation. The experimental demonstration of safety based on demonstration of absence of toxicity is in practice dependent on the nature and type of toxicity under investigation.

TOXICITY VERSUS SAFETY—EXPERIMENTAL CONCEPTS

The principle which states that there is some concentration below which all chemicals are without toxicologic effect, achieves considerable impor-

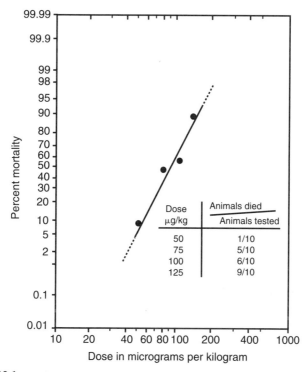

FIGURE 12.1   Lethality in male mice plotted on dose probability coordinates. The compound is hemicholinium-3, a neuromuscular paralyzing drug. The compound was administered intravenously in a tail vein. The animals were followed for 24 hr after the injection. Data were obtained in one of the author's laboratory.

tance in the design of biological tests for evaluation of safety. In fact, the existence of a threshold toxicologic dose or in other words a no-effect level or concentration of a chemical is a continuing argument as far as some forms of toxic effect are concerned although the argument, in the authors' opinion, is valid for all forms of toxicity. The controversy exists primarily because toxicity tests are conducted not only for the purpose of demonstrating the existence of toxic effects but also to estimate the limits of safety associated with the use of a compound. The problem then centers on the need to establish absence of effect beyond the level of confidence that can be achieved by ordinary experimental techniques which always involve the use of limited numbers of experimental animals.

In any attempt to establish a no-effect level or concentration of a chemical in any toxicologic test procedure, it is important to define what is meant by "effect" and the confidence that can be placed on the result of the test procedure. Basically, in order to have any toxicologic action from a chemical, there must occur some measurable phenomenon that is detrimental to the experimental animal, and it must occur within some meaningful period of time after the animal is administered the chemical. If the test animals are mice and the effect to be measured is death or any other form of toxicity of the animals, then it must be stipulated that the effect must occur within a certain period of time after administration of the chemical. The time interval could necessarily be any interval up to and including the life span of the mouse. If the effect under consideration is that of determining the influence of the chemical on the longevity of mice, the experimental time interval must necessarily be extended to the life span of the mouse. Therefore, every toxicologic experiment must necessarily define what effects are to be studied and the time interval over which they will be studied.

Since all chemicals under some conditions of use will produce toxic effects in biological sample material, it is evident that experiments usually can be designed that will show such toxic effects. In fact it is stated frequently that a good experiment is one which does demonstrate some kind of toxicity at least in the group of test animals that received the highest dose concentrations. However, even in the experiment which demonstrates a positive toxic effect the data must include adequate *negative control* information if the toxicity is to be conclusively considered as being produced by the test chemical. This means that an identical (negative control) group of animals as large or larger than the experimental group should be treated similarly to the experimental group in all respects except for omission of the chemical under test. All procedures that are performed on the test group must be performed on the control group. If a solvent is used to administer the chemical to the test group, the same solvent without the chemical should be administered to the control group. Control groups from prior experiments should not be used. These procedures should be standardized in all laboratories. In very long-term toxicity tests it also is important that a single adequate supply of the test chemical be tested and identified for purity and any presence of contaminating chemicals. The chemical should be available in sufficient quantity and properly stored for use during the entire test period. The numbers of animals used in the experimental test should be the numbers needed to yield statistically reliable results. In this manner the data from the experimental group can be ultimately compared with the data from the control group. The actual number of animals necessary to establish a cause–effect relationship is dependent on the incidence of occurrence of the toxic effect in the controls as compared to the test animals. Table 12.2 summarizes the number of animals needed in each group when there is no effect on the controls.

TABLE 12.2 Minimum Incidence of a Toxic Effect in a Series of Different Sized Groups of Animals That Can Be Considered Significant at a Probability Level of 0.025 When the Effect Is Absent in Controls and When Equal Numbers of Experimental and Control Animals Are Used[a]

Number of animals in each group	Minimum percentage incidence in experimental groups that can be regarded as significant
3	100.0
5	60.0
10	40.0
20	20.0
50	8.0
100	4.0

[a] Data from *Problems in the Evaluation of Carcinogenic Hazard from Use of Food Additives,* National Academy of Sciences—National Research Council, Publication 749, Washington, DC, 1960.

Some forms of toxicity may have also a normal occurrence in controls. In this situation in order to have an acceptable level of confidence that any positive findings in the test animals were due to the chemical, there must always be at least a specific number of examples of the toxicity in the test group greater than the number that occur in the controls. Table 12.3 lists the differences between the two groups necessary for the experimenter to have confidence that a positive finding was not due to chance in at least 95 of 100 such experiments.

In contrast to this, the good series of toxicological experiments on a chemical will demonstrate that at some lower dose no toxicity was produced. The controversial problem is whether the experiment which shows no measurable positive effect does in actuality represent a no-effect result or, in other words, a "safe" concentration or dose of the chemical. By using the same statistical concepts that were applied in the case where toxicity is demonstrated, it is apparent that, for the experiment which was conducted, the no-effect dose did indeed represent a safe dose. However, if the experiment which was conducted was performed on a relatively few animals then it would not be correct to state that the same dose was "safe" for all animals of that species unless the test included all animals. It is

TABLE 12.3   Percentage Incidence of a Normally Occurring Type of Toxicity in Control and Test Groups of Various Sizes That Can Be Considered as Significant at a Probability Level of 0.05[a]

10 Animals per group		20 Animals per group		50 Animals per group	
% Affected, control group	% Affected, test group	% Affected, control group	% Affected, test group	% Affected, control group	% Affected, test group
10	70	10	45	10	26
20	80	20	55	20	38
30	90	30	65	30	50
50	100	50	85	50	70

[a] Data from *Problems in the Evaluation of Carcinogenic Hazard from Use of Food Additives,* National Academy of Sciences—National Research Council, Publication 749, Washington, DC, 1960.

practically not feasible to test all or even a small percentage of the total number of animals in any species.

In the properly conducted test whereby negative results are obtained, it is desirable that the same test include a group of animals that show positive results for the type of toxicity under investigation. Otherwise the species that was investigated may not be fundamentally capable of showing the type of toxicity under investigation. In this case it is necessary to add to the experimental protocol a *positive control.* The positive control consists of groups of animals identical to the test group and treated in an identical manner except that a compound known to produce the type of toxicity under investigation is substituted for the test compound. Through the use of the positive control not only is the test species proven to be capable of showing the toxicity but also data will be obtained regarding the relative potency of the test compound as compared to the positive control compound.

If the objective of an experiment is to conclude that a toxic effect would not occur on more than one of a thousand test animals, then the experiment must be designed so that the confidence limits of the experimental protocol are adequate to reach such a conclusion. In any group of animals that are exposed to a given dose of a chemical and show a negative response, the limits of confidence regarding whether the experimental dose did, indeed, represent a no-effect dose must be determined by statistical methods. The limits of confidence of the experimental results are related to the number of animals in the test and control groups and the sensitivity of the experiment to demonstrate minimal amounts of toxicity. If the number of animals was high and the technical expertise was high, the confidence in the results is then high. However, elementary statistical concepts have established that even by using as many as 1000 test animals in a single test group in which no toxicity was observed, if the experimenter uses 90% confidence limits, the experiment shows that not more than 2.3 animals of the 1000 animals tested could have shown the toxic effect (Food and Drug Administration Advisory Committee on Protocols for Safety Evaluation Report, 1971). Therefore, it is generally economically infeasible to conduct toxicity tests that would establish absolute safety of many chemical entities.

The problem becomes even more complicated when the nature of the toxicity under consideration is a tremendously harmful one, such as tumorigenicity or mutagenicity, primarily because these toxicities frequently have a normal incidence of occurrence in untreated control animals. For example in the case of tests for tumorigenicity even with 1000 treated and 1000 control animals each developing 10 tumors, the experimenter can only be 95% confident that the elevation in incidence rate due to the chemical does not exceed 1%, that is, the agent could still have produced 1 additional tumor per 100 test animals. Again the demonstration of absolute safety in biologic testing methods generally is not obtainable. Extrapolation of dose–response curves outside of the range of experimental results is hazardous, and extrapolation of animal data to man in a quantitative manner is subject to great inaccuracies because of the known lack of quantitative or uniform correspondence in the toxicity of a substance for different mammalian species. When safety to man is the objective, the only rational approach to the problem is through a consideration of the nature of the toxicity in question and the application of an acceptable interpretation of benefits versus potential hazards under the conditions of intended use of the compound.

In any experimental study, the criteria which can be considered as indicative of a toxic effect in an animal as well as the duration of the experimental study can be stipulated in the design of the study. The schedule and route of exposure to the chemical can be precisely stipulated and a sufficient number of animals can be included in the experimental and control groups to ensure statistical acceptability of the study at any level of significance which the experimenter wishes to set. When these conditions are incorporated into the experiment, the results which are obtained generally will show a dose- or concentration-dependent graded response from any chemical under consideration. Such results will be obtained whether the study involves a population of single cells, such as bacteria, or a population from a species of higher animals.

TOXICITY VERSUS SAFETY—THEORETICAL CONCEPTS

Even though there are statistical and technical difficulties in establishing a no-effect dose of a chemical which would be applicable to large populations of animals, there is a theoretical basis for the existence of such a dose for all chemical agents.

Paul Ehrlich (1854–1915) initially developed the concept that in order for a chemical to produce an effect on a biological system, the chemical must react with or become "affixed" to some component of the biological system. Since the site at which the chemical compound becomes affixed was, and in most cases still is, unknown, Langley referred to this site as a "receptive substance." Currently, such sites are simply called "receptors." In those cases where receptors have been identified, the structural interaction between the drug and the receptor can be specifically defined in chemical terminology. The kinetics of the chemical receptor interaction is a simple bimolecular equilibrium reaction which is conventionally depicted as

$$C + R \rightleftarrows CR,$$

where C is the chemical and R is the receptor. This reaction obeys the Mass Law which stipulates that the concentration of the free and combined chemical is in equilibrium so that the equilibrium constant, K, for the reaction is,

$$K = \frac{[C] + [R]}{[CR]}$$

If one assumes that the concentration of the complex [CR] constitutes the stimulus that is responsible for any biologic effect, then the quantity of the complex determines the quantity of effect on the biologic system. The quantity of receptor R may be presumed to be constant in any normal biologic system. Therefore, the concentration of the chemical compound C is related directly to the concentration of CR. Hence, there must necessarily be a concentration of the chemical below which very few receptors would be occupied so that no effect is practically determinable. There must also be a range of concentrations of the chemical at which all receptors will not be occupied. Furthermore, there must be a concentration of the chemical at which for practical purposes essentially all receptors will be occupied. The theory that the quantity of the complex CR which is present at any time constitutes the stimulus that is responsible for some types of biologic effect has been questioned by the postulate that the stimulus for any biological response is produced whenever an agent molecule combines with a receptor molecule and that the rate of this combination determines the intensity of the stimulus. However, the basic concept of a chemical receptor interaction is still valid. If the affinity for any given chemical entity for a receptor is very high, then the condition for equilibrium highly favors the formation of the chemical–receptor complex which must necessarily be the case when very small quantities of toxic agents are capable of producing profound effects on a biological specimen. However, even if the affinity of a chemical for a receptor were as great as possible, it would still take a finite number of molecules of the chemical entity to occupy a significant number of receptors and therefore be capable of producing a measurable effect. The conclusion that must be reached is that there must necessarily be a quantity of chemical agent below which no biologic effect would be achieved.

CHEMICAL–BIOLOGICAL REACTIONS IN DIFFERENT SPECIES

The third principle states that cells which have similar metabolic pathways will usually be similarly affected by a given chemical entity. This concept applies not only to cells in the same species but also to similarly functioning cells in different species when appropriate pairs of species are under consideration. That is, a nerve or muscle cell in the mouse may differ in size from corresponding cells in man, but may have similar metabolic systems and functional purpose. Compounds that react with receptors which are common to either the nerve or muscle cells in one species frequently react in a similar manner with the corresponding nerve or muscle cell in the other species. This concept applies whenever the compound under test is the compound responsible for the biologic effect. However, if the compound under test is biotransformed selectively to an active compound in one species but not in another, then it is apparent that the active compound would not be present in the latter species.

When two or more mammalian species possessing functionally identical cell types, such as nerve or muscle cells, are exposed to a chemical agent, the various possibilities of achieving the same effect in the various species would be dependent on the following factors: (1) whether the receptor is present or absent, (2) whether the compound is or is not activated or inactivated in the animals, (3) whether the compound is or is not translocated to the receptor site, and (4) whether secondary substitute mechanisms are or are not available in certain species in which the affected receptor system is bypassed. Table 12.4 summarizes these possibilities and the mechanisms responsible for the occurrence or lack of occurrence of any specific

TABLE 12.4 Possible Mechanisms Responsible for the Occurrence or Lack of Occurrence of Any Specific Toxicologic Effect from Any Single Chemical Agent in Five Species Having Functionally Identical Cell Types

Functionally identical cell types	Biochemical receptor site	Toxicologic effect
Species A	Present	Present
Species A_1	Present	Present
Species A_2	Present	Absent
Species A_3	Absent	Absent
Species A_4	Absent	Present

Note. If a specific toxicologic effect can be demonstrated in a single species (Species A), then it will occur (Species A_1) or be absent (Species A_2) in other species that have the same receptor site. If the effect is absent (Species A_2), the agent has been inactivated by a biotransformation mechanism, a substitute function has taken over for the affected function, or translocation of the agent to the receptor site is blocked. In Species A_3 and A_4 the receptor site is absent but the toxicologic effect may be absent (Species A_3) or present (Species A_4). If the effect is present as in Species A_4, then either the agent has been activated by a biotransformation mechanism so that a different receptor is involved, or a secondary mechanism capable of producing the same toxicity is involved.

toxicological effect from any single agent in five species having functionally identical cell types.

Compounds having great biological interest frequently are selective in regard to their ability to affect given types of cells. When such is the case, the compound usually reacts with and inactivates some normal component (receptor) of the cell which is involved in the function of the cell. As already indicated the receptor mechanism involved frequently is not clearly definable, but if cells from two different species are affected similarly by a given chemical entity then it is probable that the same type or at least a similar type of receptor is involved in each species. Examples of systems involved in the function of cells which may be readily affected by foreign chemicals are the energy transfer systems and the systems involved in maintaining inorganic ion gradients across the cell membranes. Therefore, if two different cells are identical from a functioning standpoint, and have common biochemical regulatory mechanisms and a common receptor for the chemical agent under investigation, both cells would be similarly affected by any chemical under consideration.

There are many examples which verify this concept. An example at the molecular level is that of the reaction of arsenic with sulfhydryl groups. Such sulfhydryl groups are present in most living systems and the arsenic–sulfhydryl complex will be formed regardless of the source of the chemical group. An example at the physiological level is that certain compounds such as the barbiturates produce anesthesia equally well by an action on the central nervous system in dogs, rats, and most warm-blooded animals including man. The local anesthetic agents also block conduction of nerves whether the nerve is in the dog, cat, rat, frog, or, again, man. At a toxicologic level, carbon tetrachloride will produce similar damage to the liver in essentially all animals which have this organ. In the case of the latter examples, the receptor is not known in a chemical sense, but rather is identified as being common to the various species by virtue of the common effect produced by the chemical under consideration.

This concept achieves considerable importance when it is necessary to design an animal experiment for evaluating the toxic effects of a chemical when the data are to be extrapolated to another species such as man. It is clearly evident that the best method for the determination of the toxic effects of a chemical in man is to use man himself as the test species, or to use a species which possesses the same functional systems as man. The state of the art in toxicology at the present time is not sufficiently developed to the extent that it would be possible to predict which species is most similar to man as far as response to many chemical entities is concerned. It is very evident that there are species which are similar to man and other species which differ from man with respect to the toxic effects of individual compounds.

To carry this concept further, cells with different functions and different biochemical regulatory mechanisms may or may not be similarly affected by any given chemical entity if the action of the compound is that of affecting a biochemical regulatory mechanism. If two types of cells with no functional similarity are affected by similar amounts of a foreign chemical in a similar manner, this would be good evidence that the cellular mechanism involved in the action of the chemical was common to both types of cells. When greatly different amounts of a given chemical are necessary to produce effects on different types of cells, this would be good evidence that the mechanism of action of the chemical is different between the two examples of cells. The fact that two types of cells are not necessarily similarly affected by similar amounts of a given chemical entity is the basis of the concept of selective toxicity of chemicals. Some degree of selectivity of action of chemicals on cells is a necessary requirement for those chemical agents which are used as drug or pesticides.

The action of a chemical on a cell may be that of reacting with a component which is specific and necessary for continued function of the cell, and if the product of the reaction is not capable of functionally substituting for the role of the original component of the cell, that function of the cell is altered and/or destroyed. Whether the cell is or is not capable of continuing to survive is primarily dependent on whether other mechanisms within the cell are capable of taking over and substituting for the loss of the one or more affected mechanisms.

It is because of the selectivity of biologic action of many compounds on biochemical or physiological mechanisms that are common to cells in different species that toxicologic data obtained on animals are of value in predicting effects of the compounds in man.

In an attempt to assess the predictable value for the human of results obtained on animals, the incidence of 89 different effects caused by six drugs in three species (rats, dogs, and man) has been evaluated. From the data pertaining to the rat and dog, the occurrence or absence of each effect in man was predicted by following two rules; first, if a sign was found in both rats and dogs, it was predicted to occur in man, and second, if a sign was found in either the dog or the rat, but not in both, it was predicted that the sign would not occur in man. Since the effects of the drugs in man were already known, the number of items that were predicted correctly or incorrectly could be tabulated. Of 86 predictions for the six drugs, 26 of 38 positive predictions were correct and 38 of 48 negative predictions were correct. The average correct prediction was 74%. Predictions made on the basis of flipping a coin would be expected to yield 50% correct results, but the probability of obtaining 74% correct predictions by the coin flipping method is very small.

In this example, therefore, animal studies permitted, to some degree, prediction of drug effects in man based only on the theory that a drug action that is seen in both the rat and the dog probably involves a common physiologic mechanism that is likely to be present in the human, whereas an effect seen in only one of the two species indicates that the effect is peculiar to that species and is less likely to be present in the third species. Such evidence shows the importance of using two species in animal tests and the value of animal tests for predicting the effects of chemicals in man.

STRUCTURE–ACTIVITY FACTORS IN TOXICOLOGIC TESTS

The fourth principle states that small changes in the structure of a chemical may greatly influence the biologic action of the chemical. This principle is basically an extension of the concept that all chemical–biologic effects are the result of a physical–chemical reaction or interaction between the chemical and some component of the living system. The study of the type of chemical structure of a foreign chemical that will react with such a component is commonly referred to as the study of structure–activity relationships. Such studies have been productive in the development of drugs and pesticides. The first discovery of an example of a new chemical entity that induces biologic effects will initiate the synthesis of additional related analogs of the compound in the hopes of finding more useful or at least more effective agents capable of producing the same biologic effect. In some cases the possibilities for the synthesis of chemical analogs of effective compounds are unlimited. For example, thousands of derivatives of barbituric acid, phenothiazine, and sulfonamide-type compounds have been synthesized and tested for action on animals. Such investigations have resulted in the use of several structurally related agents as drugs to achieve a common type of biologic effect. The objective of structure–activity relationship studies is to define as precisely as possible the limits of variation in structure of a chemical nucleus which are consistent with the production of a specific biologic effect. Presumably if enough of this type of data becomes available, a hypothesis can be developed regarding the most likely structures of the receptor involved. An example of such a hypothetical formulation is the description of the active sites on the enzyme acetylcholinesterase when this enzyme is inhibited by organic phosphates or carbamates. Furthermore, the synthesis and testing of closely related homologs of known biologically active compounds occasionally result in compounds that are essentially biologically inactive on the biologic system under investigation; such information is also equally helpful in regard to the formulation of hypotheses concerning the structure of the receptor.

That small differences in chemical structures can significantly influence biologic effects of chemicals is evident in a number of examples. In pharmacology and toxicology there are several examples whereby optical isomers of single compounds or different valences on single elements have different degrees of action or even different actions. An example of the effect of optical isomerism in regard to biologic action is that shown by the drug amphetamine (racemic, B-phenylisopropylamine). This compound has several well known effects in mammals. These effects are central nervous system stimulation and stimulation of receptors which are normally innervated by the sympathetic nervous system. The d-isomer, however, is three to four times more potent than the l-isomer in regard to the action on the central nervous system, whereas the l-isomer is about two times more potent than the d-isomer in regard to its action on the heart. An example of the effect of valence on toxicity is shown by arsenic. Although the difference in the lethal toxicity of trivalent arsenic as compared to the pentavalent arsenic is not great in many mammals, the difference is considerable for lower animals and plants. The trivalent arsenites are much more lethal for protozoa, bacteria, and yeast than are the pentavalent arsenates. Chromium in the trivalent form is required for normal glucose metabolism, as an insulin cofactor; however, hexavalent chromium is carcinogenic to most animal species.

Several examples that demonstrate the fact that small changes in structure can greatly affect toxic potency have been described in regard to delayed neurotoxicity. Toxicity to the nervous system produced by several of the organophosphate and triaryl phosphate types of pesticides has been known for years. The neurotoxic action has an onset following repeated administration of low doses of the compounds. In the early stages of toxicity, animals and man show a weakness in the limbs which can progress to a state of complete paralysis. The biochemical processes that are responsible for the signs appear to be similar for all of the causative compounds; however, small changes in the structure of the compounds greatly influence the ability of the compounds to produce the neurotoxicity as shown for the following agents.

The demonstration that small changes in chemical structure may significantly influence the biologic activity of closely related chemical entities is of importance in the design of methods in toxicology. The experimental toxicologist has reservations about his confidence in being able to predict the toxicologic effect of a series of similar compounds. Rather, each compound of a series under investigation must usually be tested for all measurable effects. Also, since small changes in chemical structure can produce variations in effects, it becomes apparent that studies performed with compounds of questionable purity are valid only for that example of the test mixture. It is, indeed, rare that newly synthesized complex organic chemical agents can be said to be more than 95–98% free of impurities. Such impurities frequently are intermediates used in the synthesis procedure and therefore may be related chemically to the compound of interest, but may be solely responsible for toxicologic effects obtained in animal experimental procedures. A good example of this is the herbicide 2,4,5-trichlorophenoxyacetic acid (2,4,5T). It has been demonstrated that in the manufacture of 2,4,5T a toxic impurity was formed. The impurity was 2,3,6,7-tetrachlorodibenzodioxin (TCDD) and although it was present in the technical grade 2,4,5T only in amounts of 20 to 30 parts per million, it was found to be primarily responsible for production of birth defects in animal experiments as well as chloracne, a disfiguring skin ailment, in humans. Because of this it is necessary to eliminate TCDD in the herbicide.

DEVELOPMENT OF THE CATEGORIES OF TOXICOLOGIC TESTS

The extent to which a chemical compound is studied in the toxicology laboratory is largely dependent on the intended use of the compound. Those compounds that are intended for introduction into the human, such as drugs or food additives, obviously require extensive toxicological testing. In the case of drugs, if the compound is to be used for only short periods, i.e., a few doses, the extent of toxicological testing is different than that for drugs which are to be used over long periods of time. Another factor that determines the extent of toxicological testing is the economic importance of the chemical. Any chemical which is to be incorporated into hundreds of household preparations requires extensive toxicological testing even though it may not be intended for direct consumption by humans.

Extensive toxicological testing means that the compound is subjected to a series of individual short-term tests that are designed to detect specific types of toxicity, plus the exposure of at least two different species of animals to the compound for at least a major portion of the lifetime of the animals. If the compound eventually is to become an environmental agent, the extent of the tests involves investigations utilizing insects, fish, wildfowl, or any animal.

The generally accepted philosophy in connection with the design and conduct of toxicity tests in animals is to maintain flexibility of the protocols; however, in contrast to this philosophy in conventional practice rather rigid protocols are routinely used. The use of "fixed design" or rigid protocols in any given laboratory for each type of toxicity test has certain merits which perpetuate their use.

A rigid protocol for a toxicity test is one in which the outline of the procedure for conduct of the test is prepared so that it includes specific types and numbers of animals as test subjects, and specific routes of administration as well as dose schedules and duration of administration of the test chemical. Also, specific functional and pathologic procedures to be followed are stipulated in the test. The principal advantage of standardization of the test is that the laboratory becomes proficient in conducting the test and direct comparisons of effects produced by different compounds on essentially the same type of test can be made. Furthermore, such tests provide specific answers frequently required by governmental regulation agencies. It would, of course, be a disadvantage if the toxicologist failed to make additional observations for toxic effects which may occur during the conducting of a toxicity test but may have been unforeseen at the time the test is designed.

Over the years certain types of toxicity testing procedures have been designed, modified, and improved so that they are generally acceptable by most toxicologists. The modern toxicologist, therefore, has available a series of rather specific types of toxicological tests for the determination of the various types of toxicity. Regardless of the nature of the experimental protocol, all such tests fall into one of three major categories dependent primarily on the duration of the test. These categories are the *acute* test, the *prolonged,* test and the *chronic* test. In general, acute tests involve administration of the test chemical on one occasion. In a rare instance administration may occur on two or three closely spaced occasions. The period of observation of the test animals may be as short as a few hours, although it is usually at least 24 hr and in some cases it may be as long as a week or more. In general, prolonged tests involve administration of the test chemical on multiple occasions. The test chemical may be administered one or more times each day, irregularly as when it is incorporated in the diet, at specific times such as during pregnancy, or in some cases regularly but only at weekly intervals. Also, in the prolonged tests the experiment is usually conducted for not less than 90 days in the rat or mouse or a year in the dog. In some literature, the prolonged test is called a "subchronic toxicity test."

In contrast to the acute and prolonged types of test, the chronic toxicity tests are those in which the test chemical is administered for a substantial portion of the lifetime of the test animal. In the case of the mouse and rat, this is a period of 2 to 3 years. In the case of the dog, it is for 5 to 7 years.

These three types of toxicity tests have developed because of necessity. With all chemicals it is desirable to acquire information regarding just how much of the chemical can be given to a test animal on one or a few occasions in order to produce some minimal detectable effect, as compared to the amount necessary to produce death in the animal. The acute toxicity test serves this purpose; however, there is no assurance that the single minimal effective dose (MED) can be given to the same animal on repeated occasions without producing more intense or additional effects or in fact no measurable effect.

Table 12.5 is a general outline of the principal categories of tests commonly conducted for toxicological purposes. The table indicates that the major difference between the categories of tests is the duration of the tests. Even in the category of "special tests" the interval of time over which the animals receive the compound is frequently of considerable importance. Therefore an understanding of the factors that influence toxicity of a chemical when it is administered on a single occasion as compared to multiple occasions is fundamental to the conducting of toxicity tests.

TIME–EFFECT RELATIONSHIPS IN TOXICITY TESTS

There are examples in which a single dose of a compound given early in the life of an animal can result in considerably delayed appearance of toxicity which cannot be said to be associated with persistence of the presence of the chemical in the animal. An example is the induction of cancer appearing late in the life of the animal following administration of single doses of 3-methyl cholanthrene or 3,4-benzpyrene to the young animal. However, with the exception of carcinogenicity, chemical-induced toxicity appears to be related to the time over which exposure occurs to given concentrations of the agent.

When a single dose of a chemical alters some function of an animal, if the chemical is not given to the animal on a second occasion, any altered biochemical mechanism, function, or structure usually returns to normal after the chemical is permitted time to leave the animal by excretion or detoxication. Such an effect would be called a reversible response. If the chemical-induced damage to the tissue is so great that it is not normally repaired simply by removing the chemical, then most tissues undergo replacement of the injured tissue with new normal cells or by the development of fibrous tissue. When replacement by normal cells occurs there is no permanent injury, although such a response produced an irreversible response on the original cells. Whereas small degrees of tissue damage may not necessarily result in altered function, repeated, sufficiently frequent

TABLE 12.5   An Outline of Types of Animal Toxicologic Tests

I. Acute tests (single dose)
   A. LD_{50} determination (24-hr test and survivors followed for 7 days)
     1. Two species (usually rats and mice)
     2. Two routes of administration (one by intended route of use)
   B. Topical effects on rabbit skin (if intended route of use is topical; evaluated at 24 hr and at 7 days)

II. Prolonged tests (daily doses)
   A. Duration—3 months
   B. Two species (usually rats and dogs)
   C. Three dose levels
   D. Route of administration according to intended route of use
   E. Evaluation of state of health
     1. All animals weighed weekly
     2. Complete physical examination weekly
     3. Blood chemistry, urinalysis, hematology, and function tests performed on all ill animals
   F. All animals subjected to complete necropsy including histology of all organ systems

III. Chronic tests (daily doses)
   A. Duration—2 to 7 years depending on species
   B. Species—Selected from results of prior prolonged tests, pharmacodynamic studies on several species of animals, possible single dose human trial studies. Otherwise use two species.
   C. Minimum of two dose levels
   D. Route of administration according to intended route of use
   E. Evaluation of state of health
     1. All animals weighed weekly
     2. Complete physical examination weekly
     3. Blood chemistry, urinalysis, hematologic examination, and function tests on all animals at 3- to 6-month intervals and on all ill or abnormal animals
   F. All animals subjected to complete necropsy including histologic examination of all organ systems

IV. Special tests
   A. For potentiation with other chemicals
   B. For effects on reproduction
   C. For teratogenicity
   D. For carcinogenicity
   E. For mutagenicity
   F. For skin and eye effects
   G. For behavioral effects
   H. For immune effects

chemical-induced assault on a receptor system will generally eventually lead to altered function and grossly observable damage in that tissue. In this case the initially reversible effect can lead to irreversible changes. Generally this may be thought of as a situation whereby minimally effective doses lead to small amounts of tissue damage, and if a second dose of the chemical is given to the animal before the tissue repairs itself, the second and each subsequent dose leads to the development of added damage to the tissue. In time, the response to each dose therefore summated and resulted in intensification of the toxic effect. In such a case the repeated chemical insult to the tissue causes the toxicity to accumulate. An example of an experiment that demonstrates this accumulative concept is as follows. The local dermal toxicity of acetic acid can be determined by applying 0.1 ml of a 5% aqueous solution of acetic acid to a gauze pad and holding the pad in contact with a specific area of the shaved skin of the back of rabbits for 30 min, followed by thorough rinsing of the area with water. Separate groups of animals were treated at either daily or weekly intervals until each animal received a total of eight applications. The animals were killed 1 week following the last application of acetic acid solution. Those animals that were dosed at weekly intervals showed no gross or histologic evidence of irritant effect to the skin, whereas those animals that received the daily dose showed marked gross and histologic evidence of skin damage.

Whether a chemical compound is given on only one occasion, on many occasions, or for the lifetime of an experimental animal, the concentration–time relationship generally determines the extent of toxicity. The discussion of antidotal therapy (Chapter 11) shows that the amount of the chemical in a test specimen at any time is dependent on the rate at which the chemical enters the specimen (that is, by absorption mechanisms) versus the rate at which the chemical is eliminated from the test specimen (that is, by excretion or inactivation including storage which together constitute the mechanisms of elimination of the chemical). At any point in time, the concentration of the chemical will increase when the rate of absorption is greater than the rate of elimination of the chemical. The concentration of the chemical will be unchanged during any time interval when the absorption and elimination rates are equal. The concentration of the chemical will decline when the elimination rate exceeds the absorption rate. When repeated doses of a chemical are given to an animal at a frequency that exceeds the rate of elimination of the compound from the animal, a definite possibility exists that the concentration of the chemical can increase in the animal with time. When this occurs and the total body load of the chemical increases, the chemical is described as being "accumulative." Thus, in a sense any chemical is accumulative under the condition that it is administered to the animal at a rate which exceeds the rate of elimination of the chemical from the animal. Sufficient accumulation of the chemical in the body of an animal can lead to toxicity. This type of accumulation should be recognized as being different from the type of "accumulation of effect" previously described. The rate at which a chemical gains access to the animal is related to the dosage, the route by which it is administered, and the physical–chemical characteristics of the agent. Agents which are given by mouth or injection are, to various degrees, absorbed from the gastrointestinal tract or from the site of injection and are to various degrees distributed or translocated throughout the body. The physical–chemical factors that influence this rate of absorption and distribution (or translocation) have been discussed. Termination of action of chemicals in the body may occur simply by excretion of the compound in the expired air or via the kidneys, by biotransformation, or by selective disposition in storage (nonreceptor) areas.

THE BIOLOGICAL LIFE AND HALF-LIFE OF COMPOUNDS IN RELATION TO TOXICITY TESTS

The duration of the presence of a compound in a biological specimen is frequently referred to as the "biological life" of the compound. The conditions that influence this "biological life" may be different between species as well as between members of a species. In any experimental procedure in which only a single dose of a compound is administered to an animal, that animal will eventually elminate the compound. The process of elimination may be different between species or within different members of the same species of test animals. In the case of the compound that is eliminated solely by excretion in the urine or in the expired air, it is considerably less likely that there would be extensive differences between normal members of the species than when a compound is terminated by metabolic biotransformation processes. This is because it is highly improbable that a great difference in kidney or respiratory function can exist in normal individual animals without this condition leading to general and obvious debilitation of the animal or even the failure of the animal to survive. In contrast to this, several of the enzyme systems involved in biotransformation can be altered through genetic defects or by enzyme induction or inhibition and go unnoticed until the animal is challenged in an experiment with a suitable chemical agent.

The biological life of the compound determines the frequency of administration of the chemical in a prolonged or chronic toxicity test if accumulation of the chemical is to be avoided. From an academic point of view the ideal test would be one in which the compound under investigation was administered by a method which would enable a preselected tissue concentration to be rapidly obtained and then maintained for the duration of the study. In any prolonged toxicity study such a condition is technically and economically difficult to accomplish. From a practical point of view, it may be argued that such a condition is not even desirable. The basis of such an argument is that the usual toxicologic experiment should be performed in a manner which simulates the conditions of use of the compound by man, and it would be, indeed, rare that a human would be continuously exposed to most chemicals at a constant concentration. Even the agents which are identified as atmospheric pollutants vary in concentration from time to time depending on atmospheric conditions.

Most toxicological tests are conducted by administering the "dose" of the chemical mixed with the feed, added to the drinking water, applied to the skin as an ointment or cream or in a solvent, introduced into the breathing air, or injected by use of a hypodermic needle at periodic intervals. When the agent is added to the drinking water, the frequency of intake of the agent will vary, dependent on the animal's need and desire for water. When a compound is introduced into the atmosphere, the amount of activity and respiratory function of the animal will result in variation in the exposure and dose from time to time. When the agent is applied to the skin or injected, these conditions always involve the administration of the compound at specific intervals. Regardless of the route or method of administering a test chemical in a toxicological test, a uniform, stable, constant concentration of the chemical in the animal for the duration of the study is only rarely achieved. Since the frequency of administration is an interrupted procedure there are three possible consequences in regard to the tissue concentration of the agent.

1. If the dose is constant and the frequency of administration is sufficiently infrequent so that it is longer than the biological life of the compound, the result is a series of maximum and minimum tissue concentrations with interspaced intervals in which there will be essentially zero concentration of the agent in the tissue.

2. If the rate of administration and dose are sufficiently frequent to be shorter than the biological life, then the result is again a sequence of maximum and minimum tissue concentrations, but there will be no intervals of zero tissue concentrations. In this case if the dose and frequency of administration are not varied, as the experiment progresses each subsequent dose would be expected to produce a maximum tissue concentration which is greater than that produced by the previous dose. This is because the maximum tissue concentration is a result of the summation of the concentration of the residual chemical from the previous dose, plus the concentration

that is created by each subsequent dose. It is now apparent that in time, unless the quantity of each dose is decreased or the interval between administration of the doses of the compound is lengthened, the chemical will in time progressively accumulate in the test animal. In actual practice the amount of accumulated chemical in the animal is self-limiting because of mechanisms which will be described. However, in this manner, an animal eventually can accumulate a sufficient concentration of the chemical to result in toxicity.

3. If the rate of administration and dose of the agent are modified during a prolonged or chronic experiment so that the dose administered at any interval is just adequate to replace that portion of the previous dose which was eliminated from the animal during the interval between doses, the result in regard to tissue concentration of the agent is a fluctuating maximal and minimal concentration which is synchronized with the frequency of dosing. At this time an average overall steady state of the body load of the chemical is maintained. Because the rate of administration equals the rate of elimination, the maximal and minimal tissue concentrations would not vary and the agent would not accumulate in the animal. This situation can be accomplished in an experimental animal by periodic analytical monitoring of the tissue concentrations. It also can be approximated when sufficient information on the biological life of the compound becomes available.

It is common practice to determine the biologic "half-life" of a compound whenever an analytical method for the compound is available. The biologic half-life of a compound in an animal is that interval of time in which one-half of the compound present in the body is eliminated from the body. In actual practice the biologic half-life is determined by measurement of the interval of time during which the concentration of the compound in the body following a single dose of the compound decreases to half of any given concentration. This is done at a time when absorption of the compound is complete.

The concept of the existence of the biologic half-life of a compound in the body is generally valid because most of the elimination mechanisms result in an elimination of a constant fraction of the total amount of the chemical in the body with each equal interval of time. In other words, as the concentration of the compound in the body increases its rate of elimination from the body increases. This is basically the condition developed by first order kinetics, that is, at any particular moment the rate of elimination is a finite figure, but as the concentration of the chemical in the body changes, the rate of elimination changes. Although the biologic half-life is obtained by administering a single dose of the compound to an animal and measuring the time required for a tissue concentration to decline to 50%

of its initial concentration, the result obtained is valid only if the measurement is made at a time when absorption of the chemical from its site of administration is complete. However, some compounds are eliminated at a rate which is independent of the concentration of the compound in the body at least until low concentrations are involved. In this case, and according to the definition of a biologic half-life as stated above, the half-life would be different when different concentrations of the chemical were involved.

Additional factors can influence the biologic half-life of certain compounds when they are given on multiple occasions. For example, if a compound is detoxified in the animal by enzymatic biotransformation it is not uncommon to find that the compound "induces" the enzyme responsible for its own detoxification. When this occurs the rate of termination of action of the compound is changed and consequently the half-life of the compound would be changed.

The pharmacologist and the physician, in the course of using drugs, are primarily interested in establishing a fixed dose and a dosage schedule that will create a specifically optimal concentration of a drug in the human. Such a concentration of the drug would presumably be that which would achieve the therapeutic objective and avoid any covert toxic effect. Such a concentration is referred to as the "effective drug concentration." With many, if not most, drugs, the biologic half-life and the rate constant for elimination of the drug from the body are known. When such information is available, if it is assumed that the absorption rate of the drug follows zero order kinetics (that is, there is a constant rate of absorption and that absorption is complete during the time interval between doses) and that the rate of elimination is according to first order kinetics (that is, it is an exponential rate of elimination), it then is possible to predict by the use of suitable mathematical formulas the optimal dose, the number of doses, and the interval between doses that would be required to achieve the effective drug concentration. The equations for this purpose can be found in the textbook references cited in Chapter 15.

Some prolonged and chronic toxicity studies are performed on compounds under conditions for which there is no known method for analytical measurement of the concentration of the compound in the tissue. Furthermore, even when chemical analytical methods are available, distribution of a test compound would have to be known or simple monitoring of blood would not reflect the extent of accumulation of the compound in other compartments of the animal.

In contrast to the need of the pharmacologist to achieve a "therapeutic" and presumably constant concentration of a drug in the body, the toxicologist seeks to ascertain how to produce, as well as how to prevent, the occurrence of toxicity. The biologic half-life of a compound does not supply information regarding either a therapeutic or a toxicologic effect. However, since toxicologic effect is fundamentally related to concentration of the chemical at the effector sites, knowledge of the half-life could be used under some conditions to determine whether accumulation of the compound would occur. If accumulation of the compound did occur and the plateau that was finally reached was above the threshold for the occurrence of toxicity, then one would expect toxicity to occur at a time that could be predicted from the dose, the frequency of administration, and the half-life of the compound. However, if a single dose of a compound was great enough to produce some form of toxicity which outlasts the biological life of the compound, then toxicity would accumulate from repeated doses of the compound even though the doses were separated by a period of time greater than the biological life of the compound in the animal. That is, at least from a theoretical standpoint toxicity could accumulate without accumulation of the chemical at the receptor sites in the animal. Because of the importance in toxicology of the relationships between the biologic half-life when it is used as a measure of accumulation of a chemical and the toxicologic effects as they are manifested because of accumulation of the chemical, this subject is considered in greater detail in the following paragraphs.

The biologic half-life of a compound has been shown to be a major factor that determines whether a compound will accumulate in an experimental subject upon repeated exposure to the chemical. Since accumulation of a chemical is one mechanism that leads to elevated concentrations of a chemical in a biologic system, and since all toxicities are concentration related, the rate of onset and development of toxicity will be related directly to the rate of accumulation, and thus the half-life, of the compound in an experimental animal. In contrast, the rate of recovery of a biologic system from a chemical-induced toxicity may or may not parallel the rate of elimination of the chemical from the animal. In other words, the "half-life of recovery from a toxicologic effect" does not necessarily parallel the biologic half-life, which is a measure of the rate of disappearance of the chemical from the animal. Rather, the half-life of a toxicologic effect is a function of the degree to which the effect is or is not reversible. This concept applies to all forms of toxicity, including carcinogenesis, teratogenesis, and mutagenesis, and not just various types of degenerative organ toxicity, since in every type of toxic effect the initial chemical insult must involve some finite degree of damage to a cell. Such damage can be sufficient to be permanent and self-perpetuating, as in mutagenicity and/or carcinogenicity, or insufficient so that regeneration of the cell to normal takes place.

If it is assumed that all reversible toxicologic effects result from derangement, short of death, of a biologic system as a result of an unfavorable exposure to a chemical, then once the chemical has been removed from the deranged system, it will return to its normal function state either (1) immediately, because the effect is readily reversible and dependent only on the presence and concentration of the chemical, or (2) delayed, because the effect is either slowly reversible or nonreversible so that it persists beyond the time when the chemical can be detected in the biologic system. In the situation for which recovery from an effect is immediate (or at least rapid), the direct relation between a declining concentration and recovery is easily comprehended. In the situation for which recovery is delayed, several mechanisms may be involved and these mechanisms are collectively referred to in pathology as the "regeneration process." Whenever a biologic cell is damaged short of death, regardless of the cause of the damage, the cell may undergo the process of "regeneration," which only means that it returns to normal both functionally and structurally.

The mechanisms responsible for regeneration of damaged cells are not clearly definable, but for purposes of this discussion, the mechanisms are time dependent and can be demonstrated by the following example. When ethyl alcohol is administered to animals or humans in an adequately large dose, one effect of the alcohol is that of causing the deposition of abnormal amounts of fat in the liver cells. The fat can be seen in histologic sections of the liver, and can be determined analytically from a sample of the liver. The alcohol disappears from the body (by metabolic and excretory mechanisms), and in time the accumulated fat disappears from the liver; however, this latter process involves considerably more time than the time involved in losing the alcohol. If additional exposure to alcohol occurs before the cells have regenerated to normal, additional fat will be deposited in the liver. Thus the toxicity, manifested as fat deposition, can accumulate under conditions in which the alcohol does not accumulate. Furthermore, if the rate of regeneration of the cells was measured analytically in the absence of additional exposure to alcohol, it would be possible to determine quantitatively the time required for the tissue to regenerate to a degree equal to 50% improvement. This figure would represent the "half-life for recovery from the toxic effect" (hereafter referred to as the "half-life of the toxic effect"). If the rate of regeneration was exponential, that is, related directly to the total amount of fat present, the half-life of the toxic effect would be a fixed figure, regardless of the degree of accumulation of fat in the liver. However, if the rate of regeneration was linear and independent of the amount of fat in the liver, then the half-life of the toxic effect would vary with variations in the degree of liver damage.

Thus a general concept appears to be valid whenever exposure to a chemical is repetitive. The concept is that if the initial exposure to a chemical is sufficient to reach or exceed a threshold of some form of toxicity, and if the half-life of the toxic effect exceeds the biologic half-life of the chemical, then it is not necessary for the chemical to accumulate in the animal in order for the toxic effect to accumulate. However, if the animal is exposed to a chemical on repeated occasions such that the interval between exposures is sufficiently less than the biologic half-life of the compound and accumulation of the chemical occurs, as the accumulated concentrations of the chemical approach the threshold of producing a toxicity, that toxicity would become evident. Then, if the half-life of the toxic effect is greater than the biologic half-life of the chemical, the amount of toxicity would progressively approach a plateau.

Figure 12.2 diagrammatically presents an example of the relationship between accumulation of a chemical and accumulation of its toxic effect. In the figure, a readily absorbed compound is administered to an animal

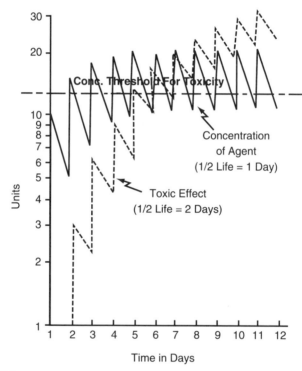

FIGURE 12.2   Diagrammatic representation of relationship between the rate of accumulation of a chemical and the rate of accumulation of a toxic effect from the chemical. The chemical is administered daily at a uniform dose schedule and its biologic half-life is 1 day. The half-life of the toxic effect is 2 days. Both the concentration and the toxicity are in arbitrary units.

at a uniform daily dosage rate which is adequate to produce a whole-body maximum concentration of 10 units. The biologic half-life of the compound is 1 day, and the threshold concentration for the occurrence of toxicity is 12 units. Thus the toxic effect occurs whenever the concentration of the agent exceeds 12 units. The half-life of the toxic effect is 2 days. Elevating the threshold of toxicity would shift the cumulative toxicity curve to the right. Lowering the threshold of toxicity would shift the cumulative toxicity curve to the left. Also, increasing the biologic half-life of the chemical or increasing the half-life of the toxic effect would shift the toxic effect curve in the figure to the left, whereas decreasing the biologic half-life of the chemical or the half-life of the toxic effect would shift the toxic effect curve in the figure to the right.

Under the practical conditions of exposure of humans to chemicals in their occupations or in their environment, chemicals that have short biologic half-lives are less likely to accumulate than chemicals that have longer biologic half-lives. In a similar manner, chemicals that produce toxicities with short half-lives are less likely to produce accumulated toxicity than chemicals that produce toxicities with long half-lives. A relatively safe chemical would be one that had a short biologic half-life and produced toxicities that were readily reversible, i.e., it would produce only those toxicities that have short half-lives.

A classical experimental method for measuring the cumulative effect of compounds orally administered to animals is described below. The method involves comparing the 1-dose LD_{50} with the 90-dose LD_{50}. The 90-dose LD_{50} was selected because there is experimental evidence which shows that 90-day studies in rats and dogs involving daily dosing of the animals showed results that were similar to corresponding lifetime studies in these species for a wide range of compounds (except for cancer). The procedure determines the 1-dose LD_{50} when the compound was given by stomach tube to groups of rats. The 90-dose LD_{50} was determined by addition of appropriate concentrations of the compound in the feed for the animals. Groups of rats were fed different concentrations of the test compound for 90 days. The range of doses was sufficiently large so that some of the animals died during the 90-day interval. All surviving animals were followed for a minimum of 2 weeks after the 90-day period. The dose in the 90-dose study was expressed as mg/kg/day as calculated from measured feed consumption. The ratio of the 1-dose LD_{50} to the 90-dose LD_{50} is a measure of cumulative effect of the compound. This ratio expressed as a quotient is called the "chronicity factor" for the compound. By definition, therefore, a chronicity factor of 90 would mean that the compound was absolutely cumulative; that is, the 90-day LD_{50} in mg/kg/day equals 1/90th of the 1-dose LD_{50}. The chronicity factor is greater than 2.0 for compounds that are relatively cumulative in their effects and less than 2.0 for compounds that show little cumulative effect. Warfarin (3-α-phenyl-β-acetylethyl-4-hydroxy-coumarin), an antiocoagulant drug, was found to have a chronicity factor of 2.0. The chronicity factor for potassium cyanide (mixed with the feed) was 0.04, suggesting that the presence of feed along with each dose markedly protected the animal from the effect of potassium cyanide. The test is not applicable to all chemicals since some compounds mixed with feed result in poor acceptance of the feed by the animals.

In the process of designing prolonged and chronic biological tests for detection of toxicity, it is therefore highly desirable to be able to obtain some information regarding cumulative effects of the compound and on the biologic half-life and the effect of repeated dosing on the half-life of the compound which is under investigation. When prolonged 90-day experiments are conducted at a fixed dose schedule, unless that dose schedule is adjustly appropriately to accommodate for the biologic half-life of the compound, the experiment will eventually result either in progressive accumulation of the compound in the animal until a steady state is reached or in repeated challenges to the animals with intervals of absence of exposure to the chemical that is under investigation. Since toxicity in general is always related to the concentration of the chemical at the effector sites, the foregoing discussion indicates that some compounds studied under the conditions of two different dose frequencies could lead to different conclusions about the quantity of the chemical necessary to produce any type of toxicity, as well as the quantity of the chemical which would be considered as "safe."

Some prolonged and chronic toxicity studies are performed utilizing so-called "maximally tolerated doses" in animals. The highest dose which permits the animal to survive without effect is the dose which is called the maximally tolerated dose. The determination of the maximally tolerated dose is usually experimentally derived from short-term studies. This involves exposing groups of animals to various fixed doses and fixed frequency (unless the dose is incorporated in the feed of the animal) schedules from 10 days to a few weeks. The animals are observed for the interval of the test and are killed and examined for evidence of abnormal or toxicological changes which may be the result of administering the chemical to the animal. From this experiment a dose and a method of administration of the dose are obtained which permit the animal to survive in an apparently normal condition. The animals in that group which received the next highest dose of the chemical must of course have shown toxicity as a result of administration of the chemical if the objective of the experiment is to determine the maximally tolerated dose.

SUMMARY OF PRINCIPLES INVOLVED IN TOXICITY TESTS

The foregoing discussion demonstrates that certain prerequisite information is desirable before the toxicologist can develop an intelligent program for testing the toxicity of any compound. This consists of at least the following three types of information. The first concerns a knowledge of the nature and chemical purity as well as the physical–chemical characteristics of the compound. On many occasions, the compound of interest is that which would be available commercially rather than the absolutely pure compound, merely because the pure agent would only rarely be available for general use. Hence most toxicity studies consist of the toxicological evaluation of a mixture of chemicals of which one constitutes the majority of the mixture. From this information, the toxicologist can estimate, on the basis of prior knowledge and from the published literature, the possible nature of action of the compound and even perhaps the degree of expected potency of the compound. The physical–chemical characteristics of the compound, such as solubility in various solvents, dissociation constants, and stability, will aid the toxicologist in determining the route by which the compound can be administered to experimental animals and will indicate how the compound will be distributed in the various tissues of the animals as well as how the compound will be eliminated from the animal.

The second type of prerequisite information which is highly desirable concerns an analytical method for quantitative estimation of the chemical in biological sample material. When such a method is available, the rate of absorption from various routes of administration can be determined. The biologic half-life of the compound can be determined. Dosage schedules can be designed to preclude excessive accumulation of the compound in the animal in prolonged or chronic tests. Effects observed in the animal can be related to tissue concentrations of the compound. The mechanism of elimination can be determined and predictions can be developed regarding the most suitable test animals species for the subsequent toxicological tests. If the compound is one which is biotransformed in the animal, the rate and products of biotransformation can be estimated.

The third type of information desirable before toxicological tests are conducted concerns any prior biologic studies on the compound or closely related compounds. Such information will give the toxicologist an estimate of the nature of toxicologic effects that may be anticipated in his studies. Compounds that produce specific organ damage, such as damage to the liver, kidney, or intestine, will suggest that certain biologic and chemical function tests should be incorporated early in the toxicological testing protocols. The duration of action of single as well as multiple doses of structurally related compounds may be of value as an indication of the degree of reversibility or irreversibility of the effects of the compound.

The objective of toxicological testing is to evaluate the relative potential of a compound for producing harm to biological tissue. The procedures therefore necessarily involve the use of species of animals in which the amount of the compound that is given to some of the animals is sufficiently great so that distinct toxicity is produced. The procedures involved also necessitate the administration of the compound in sufficiently small amounts so that no detectable effect results. In the most strict sense, even then, the data that are obtained have some extrapolative value to estimate the potential toxicity of the compound in other species of animals that are at least in a similar category in the biological kingdom. Although relative harmfulness may be thought of as a reciprocal of safeness of a compound, the science of toxicology has not reached the degree of perfection so that any compound can be proven to be absolutely safe under all conditions of use in essentially any population. Safeness of a compound is contingent always on the condition of use of the compound and can be expressed only in terms of the probabilities that harm would not occur. For every condition of use of a compound, an evaluation must be eventually made which stipulates the frequency, the degree, and the type of harm that will be acceptable if a compound is to be used.

After completion of animal toxicity tests, only the use of the compound by man will reveal any subtle and unforeseen toxicity. Therefore, toxicological testing is not complete until the compound has stood the test of time and use in the hands of man. Even then, when the compound is used by man, unless there is adequate follow-up and recording of untoward effects from the compound, it may become generally recognized as safe without adequate data to support that contention.

The procedures for animal toxicity testing have proven to be a successful means of evaluating the harmfulness of compounds for man. When various types of toxicity occur in man that were not observed in proper animal tests, a retrospective review of the animal data reveals that the studies performed or the species tested was not appropriate for the type of toxicity which was revealed in man. Usually when a toxicity becomes evident in man and the compound then is taken back to the laboratory and tested in the proper species of animals, positive results are seen in the experimental animal. There is no doubt that the early and adequate toxicological evaluation of chemicals in animals clearly warns about the harmfulness associated with the use of a compound and thereby prevents distinctly harmful compounds from becoming generally available. Thus in modern society no compound should be made available for general human use without appropriate toxicological evaluation by accepted methodology.

CHAPTER **13**

Toxicologic Testing Methods

In general all toxicity testing methods can be divided into two categories. The first category consists of tests that are designed to evaluate the
overall effects of compounds on experimental animals. The individual tests
in this category differ from each other basically in regard to the duration
of the test and the extent to which the animals are evaluated critically for
general toxicity. The tests are identified as acute, prolonged, and chronic
toxicity tests.

The second category of tests consists of those tests that are designed to
evaluate in detail specific types of toxicity. The prolonged and chronic tests
do not detect all forms of toxicity but they may reveal some of the specific
toxicities and indicate the need for more detailed studies. Also, the intended
use of a compound may require that an estimate of the order of safety
from certain specific toxicities be investigated. The second category of
toxicity tests has been developed to fill these needs. Examples of specific
toxicity tests are: (1) those that determine the effects on the fetus in a
pregnant animal, that is, teratogenic tests, (2) tests to determine effects on
reproductive capacity of the animals, that is, reproduction tests, (3) tests
to determine effects on the genetic code system, that is, mutagenic tests,
(4) tests to determine the ability of agents to produce tumors, that is, tests
for tumorigenicity and carcinogenicity, (5) tests to determine local effects
of agents when they are applied directly to the skin and eyes, (6) tests to
determine the effect of agents on various behavior pattern of animals, that

is, behavioral or neurotoxicity tests, and (7) tests to determine the effects on the immune system, that is, immunotoxicity tests. These tests will be described in the order listed.

Certain technical and procedural factors are common to the conduct of all types of toxicity studies on experimental animals. These are the preparation of a suitable form of the chemical for administration purposes, the selection of the route or routes of administration to be used, and the species of animals to be used in the study. All of these factors are collectively considered since each influences the others.

It is essential that the chemical and physical characteristics of any test material used in a toxicology study whether actue, prolonged, or chronic be thoroughly evaluated for its composition. The purity of the material and its major contaminant should be thoroughly evaluated both from the standpoint of the initial chemical or mixture and from the standpoint of its durability throughout the testing protocol. In repeat studies, the stability of the chemical should be understood and the products of degradation evaluated because of their own unique toxicity or their ability to alter the toxicity of the test material. Chemical analyses should be conducted before the initiation of the prolonged study to ensure that the test material is stable for the period of its intended use. This evaluation can be conducted concurrently with the study but detection of instability during the study could invalidate the results. If the material is stored only under certain conditions, e.g., frozen storage, special arrangements for storage should be made. Instability of the test material may result in lower than expected doses and the exposure of the animal to degradation products may occur. Methodologies need to be developed for evaluating the compound and/or its metabolites in the carrier whether it is mixed with feed or in an aerosol.

In order to formulate a preparation of a compound for administration to animals, it is desirable to take advantage of the solubility characteristics of the compound. Water or physiological saline (0.9% NaCl in water) is always the solute of choice since these solvents permit administration by all routes. When this is not possible because of solubility limitations, it is necessary to resort to the use of vegetable oils such as corn oil or even organic solvents, of which propylene glycol is commonly used. Whenever possible the use of suspensions or emulsions should be avoided except for oral administration. Regardless of the route of administration, the volume required to administer a given dose is limited by the size of the animal that is used. It is desirable to keep the volume of each dose uniform within and between groups of animals. When rats or mice are used the volume administered by the oral route should not exceed 0.005 ml per gram of animal. Even when aqueous or physiological saline solutions are used for parenteral injection the volumes that are tolerated are limited, although such solutions are ordinarily thought of as being innocuous. The intravenous LD_{50} of distilled water in the mouse is approximately 0.044 ml per gram and that of isotonic saline is 0.068 ml per gram of mouse.

When a compound is to be administered by inhalation, special techniques for generating test atmospheres are necessary. Dose estimation becomes very complicated. The methods usually involve aerosolization or nebulization of fluids containing the compound. If the agent to be tested is a fluid that has an appreciable vapor pressure, it may be administered by passing air through the solution under controlled temperature conditions. Under this condition, dose is estimated from the volume of air inhaled per unit time, the temperature of the solution, and the vapor pressure of the agent involved. Gases are metered from reservoirs. When particles of a solution are to be administered, unless the particle size is less than 2 μm the particles will not reach the terminal alveolar sacs in the lungs. A variety of apparatuses and chambers exists to perform studies for detecting effects of irritants or other toxic endpoints when they are administered by inhalation.

The simplest method of administering an agent to animals is via the oral route, either by intubation or by incorporating the agent in the feed. Admixture of the test agent in the feed is precluded if it is unstable or if it reacts with the components of the feed to any degree that would alter the properties of the compound. Also, in some cases the presence of a test chemical in the feed may affect the acceptability of the feed by the test animals. The approximate quantity of feed consumed daily by most species of animals used in toxicity tests is known. Liquids or solids that are soluble in water may be added to the drinking water of the test animals. In each case the daily dose is calculated by monitoring the daily intake of feed or water.

It previously has been indicated that, with the exception of acute toxicity tests, most tests are conducted for the purpose of determining the nature of any toxicity that can be produced by repeated dosing of animals over an extended period of time and for estimating the degree of safety of a material for man. Some guidelines should be considered whenever experimental studies are contemplated.

1. Wherever practical or possible, use one or more species that biologically handle the material qualitatively as similarly as possible to man. For this, metabolism, absorption, excretion, storage, and other physiological effects should be considered.

2. Where practical, use several dose concentrations on the principle that all types of toxicologic and pharmacologic action in man and animals are dose-related. The only exception to this should be the use of a single, maximum dosage if the material is relatively nontoxic; this concentration

should be a sufficiently large multiple of that which is attainable by the maximum applicable hazard exposure route, and should not be physiologically impractical.

3. Effects produced at higher doses (within the practical limits discussed above) are useful for delineating mechanism of action, but for any material and adverse effect, some dose concentration exists for man or animal below which this adverse effect will not appear. This biologically insignificant concentration can and should be set by use of a proper safety factor (uncertainty factor) and competent scientific judgment.

4. Statistical tests for significance are valid only for the experimental units (e.g., either litters or individuals) that have been mathematically randomized among the dosed and concurrent control groups. It is to be understood that statistical significance may be of little or no biological importance and, conversely, that important biological trends should be further examined even in the absence of statistical significance.

5. Effects obtained by one route of administration to test animals are not a priori applicable to effects by another route of administration to man. The routes chosen for administration to test animals should, therefore, be the same as those by which man will be exposed. Thus, for example, food additives for man should be tested by admixture of the material in the diet of animals.

It is therefore apparent that there are no fixed rules regarding the selection of specific species of animals for toxicologic tests. In the absence of some specific reason for the use of relatively expensive species, such as nonhuman primates, dogs, or cats, most toxicity studies are performed on rats, mice, guinea pigs, and rabbits; these animals are relatively inexpensive, readily obtainable, and easily handled, and there is a considerable amount of toxicologic information regarding the effects of most chemical entities on these species.

Details of the tests summarized in this chapter as well as the importance of care and maintenance of experimental animals are beyond the scope of this chapter but can be found in the textbooks listed in Chapter 15.

ACUTE TOXICITY TESTS

The single test that is conducted on essentially all chemicals that are of any biologic interest is the acute toxicity test. The test consists of administering the compound to the animals on one occasion. The purpose of the test is to determine the symptomatology consequent to administration of the compound and to determine the order of lethality of the compound.

The initial procedure is to perform a series of range-finding doses of the compound in a single species. This necessitates selection of a route of administration, preparation of the compound in a form suitable for administration by the slected route, and selection of an appropriate species. It has already been stated that the intended use of the compound suggests the most suitable route for the initial tests. However, even if the intended use of the compound does not involve the oral or parenteral routes, at least the oral route is used in addition to other routes for comparative purposes with other related compounds and for estimating the use of this route for subsequent, more extensive and prolonged toxicity studies. It is apparent that the data which will be obtained are limited to those routes of administration that are used in the experimental procedure. The compound may be less toxic following oral administration than it is following intramuscular administration because it is not absorbed or is poorly absorbed from the gastrointestinal tract or is detoxified by passage through the liver following absorption from the gut. Lethality following intraperitoneal administration may be less than that following intravenous administration as a result of liver detoxication of the compound or by enterohepatic cycling of the compound unless the toxic effect of the compound is localized in the liver.

Essentially all initial, acute toxicity tests are performed on either rats or mice because of their low cost, their availability, and the fact that abundant reference toxicologic data for most compounds are available for these species. However, when subsequent studies are to be performed on other species such as rabbits or guinea pigs, a procedure similar to that used with rats or mice is followed to obtain an estimation of the order of lethal toxicity in these additional species of animals. Regardless of the species selected, all test animals should be in a state of good health and should be observed for a period of time (1 week for rats or mice, 3 to 4 weeks for dogs) in the laboratory or central animal quarters prior to the tests.

The classical sequence for determining the acute toxicity of a new compound consists of an initial dose-range-finding experiment, a subsequent experiment to narrow the range of effective doses for measurement of lethality, and finally a definitive experiment for establishing the dose–response curve for lethality.

The initial rough dose-range-finding experiment involves selecting doses based on suspected toxicity which is obtainable only from a knowledge of the structure of the compound and prior information on the toxicity of structurally related compounds. When rats or mice are used, only two animals are used for each dose. By using logarithms of the dose, a range of doses is experimentally determined that will produce death versus no effect or minimal effects. The animals are observed for a minimum of 24 hr. If the animals appear to be healthy at the end of 24 hr, they are set aside and observed at daily intervals for at least 1 week for appearance of delayed toxicity.

A second series of tests then is performed on the same species using four animals in each test group in an attempt to narrow the range of doses so that data are obtained for doses that produce death in less than all of the members of a high-dose group and at least signs of intoxication in a low-dose group. The animals are followed as in the initial experiment.

When the data from the preliminary dose-finding tests are obtained, the final experiment is performed. A total number of animals of similar body weight and of the same sex or equal numbers of both sexes are selected and assigned randomly to test and control groups so that each group contains 10 animals (rats or mice). Each group is administered different doses of the formulation which previously has been estimated to produce between 10 and 90% mortality. The sequence of effects following the administration of the compound has already been observed so that time of onset of signs as well as time of death or time of recovery from signs is recorded accurately. The LD_{50} is then statistically determined according to methods described in Chapter 2.

When animals are exposed to the varying concentrations of the test compound via inhalation, the lethal concentration required to produce death in 50% of the animals is determined. During the test, the duration of exposure is always kept constant. Usually the experiment involves a 4-hr exposure period and the animals then are observed for 2 weeks after exposure. The LCT_{50} (lethal concentration time) is then determined. The LCT_{50} in this case is the concentration of the test agent which is required to kill 50% of the animals when exposure is for 4 hr.

A list of typical types of effects that may be observed or elicited during experimental determination of the acute toxicity of a compound on rats and mice is found in Table 13.1.

From these data the experienced toxicologist can arrive at certain conclusions regarding the site and mechanisms of action of compounds undergoing the test.

When suitably extensive observations are made of the signs of animals used for acute toxicity tests, it is possible to estimate the minimal symptomatic or toxic dose, the maximal tolerated dose for which the animals recover completely from all effects of the chemical, and the dose that produces no effect in the test species. On the basis of such information, estimations of the duration of action of single doses may be made for use in subsequent repeated dose types of toxicity tests.

In the acute toxicity study, every effort is made to obtain information that can be used for subsequent prolonged toxicity studies. If subsequent, more prolonged experiments are planned using rats or dogs, the acute test

TABLE 13.1 Physical and Observational Examination of Animals in Toxicity Studies

Activity
  Dec locomotor activity
  Inc locomotor activity
  Jumping
Bizarre reaction
  Circus movements
  Aimless wandering
  Backward movements
  Waltzing
  Nuzzling
  Licking compartment walls
  Shovel-nose movements
  Glassy-eyed stare
  Circling movements
Phonation
  Inc phonation
  Dec phonation
  Abnormal phonation
Sensitivity to pain
  Inc sensitivity
  Dec Sensitivity
  Analgesia
Sensitivity to sound
  Inc sensitivity
  Dec sensitivity
  Reactivity
Sensitivity to touch
  Inc sensitivity
  Dec sensitivity
  Pinnal reflec depr
  Pinnal reflec abs
Social interaction
  Inc exploratory behavior
  Dec exploratory behavior
  Inc rearing frequency
  Inc speed of rearing
  Dec rearing frequency
  Dec rearing height
Abnormal tail
  Rigid tail
  Straub tail
  Limp tail
Aggressive behavior
  Inc—specied toward same species
  Dec—species
  Inc—people toward experimenters
  Dec—people

Ataxia
Convulsions
  Tonic convulsions
  Clonic convulsions
  Mixed convulsions
  Subconvulsions
  Subconvulsive movements
Muscle tone
  Inc muscle tone—trunk
  Dec muscle tone—trunk
  Inc muscle tone—limbs
  Dec muscle tone—limbs
Paralysis
Somatic response
  Inc preening
  Dec preening
  Rubbing nose
  Inc scratching
  Dec scratching
  Writhing
Postural reflexes
  Placing reflex depr
  Placing reflex abs
  Grasping reflex depr
  Grasping reflex depr
  Righting reflex depr
  Righting reflex abs
Prostration
  Prostration
  Loss of consciousness
Tremors
  Tremors—rest and movement
  Tremors—movement only
Exophthalmos
Eye irritation
  Eye opacity
  Blinking—excessive
  Iritis
Corneal reflex
  Corneal reflex abs
  Corneal reflex depr
Lacrimation
Nystagmus
Pupillary light reflex
  Pupillary reflex abs
  Pupillary reflex depr
Photophobia

(*continues*)

TABLE 13.1   (*Continued*)

Pupil size	Dec respiration depth
Mydriasis	Irregular respiration
Miosis	Cardiac
Defecation	Heart rate
Inc defecation	Pulse
Dec defecation	Nasal discharge
Diarrhea	Body temp
Bloody stool	Inc rectal temp
Salivation	Dec rectal temp
Salivation	Cyanosis
Dry mouth	Motor deficit
Urination	Mot def inclined strip
Inc urination	Mot def roa-rod
Dec urination	Mot def horizontal wire
Hematuria	Piloerection
Apnea	Death
Dyspnea	No effect
Respiration	Special Functional tests
Inc respiration rate	Conditioned-avoidance behavior
Dec respiration rate	Conditioned-reflex response
Inc respiration depth	

Note. Abbreviations used: dec, decreased; inc, increased; depr, depressed; abs, absent.

should be conducted first on rats; from these data an estimate of a single nonlethal dose of the compound can be determined for dogs. In this manner similarities and dissimilarities in signs between species can be evaluated. Usually chemical methods for determining the concentration of a new chemical in biologic tissue are not available, but if an analytical method is available and an experiment is conducted on dogs some information on distribution of the chemical in the various body fluid compartments and organs can be obtained; this information can be correlated with signs. It is possible also to determine the route of excretion and the half-life of the compound in the animal, provided the analytic methodology is sufficiently specific and sensitive.

The LD_{50} values should be reported in terms of the duration over which the animals were observed. That is, if the test animals were observed for 24 hr after the administration of the compound the results represent a 24-hr LD_{50}. Whenever the interval of time is not indicated, it is generally assumed that the animals were followed for 24 hr. Occasionally it is desirable to follow the animals for periods considerably longer than 14 days. For example, it is well known that tricresyl phosphate will produce a neurological syndrome in animals after a single dose but only after an interval of 10 to 14 days. Carcinogenic compounds and those compounds used in the treatment of carcinoma frequently show delayed toxicities and delayed deaths. Although single dose 24-hr or 7-day LD_{50} values usually can be determined for such compounds, the quantity of the compound required to produce short-term deaths is large and has little practical value for comparison purposes with other similarly acting compounds. Whenever deaths are delayed, the compound is strongly suspected of having the potential for accumulation when repeated doses are given at a daily rate. Whenever such a compound is to be studied in prolonged types of studies, it is useful to determine the effects and lethality of several daily doses. Such an LD_{50} can be obtained by administering four or five daily doses and then following the animals for 4 weeks. At least two different routes of administration are used on groups of four animals for each test done. In this manner the accuracy of estimating the range of doses required in prolonged toxicity studies is increased greatly.

In vitro replacement methods for acute toxicity testing are difficult to define. A number of *in vitro* strategies have been suggested to replace whole animal acute toxicity testing; however, none have been accepted for regulatory purposes. A variety of procedures have been suggested to reduce the number of animals necessary and to refine protocols to minimize pain and suffering of animals. Included among these protocols are a variety of modified LD_{50} tests, e.g., approximate lethal dose method, the up-and-down method, the British Society of Toxicology Protocol, and the fixed dose procedure.

Although many regard the issue of alternative methods for animal testing as no more than animal rights activism that is solely based on humanitarian reasons, animal testing nonetheless continues to be widely debated. There are three recognized alternatives, the so-called 3 R's: Reduction, Refinement, and Replacement. Reduction of the number of animals used in testing and refinement of existing testing methods to minimize the pain and suffering of animals represent the short-term objectives. Replacement of animal testing with nonanimal based methods, e.g., *in vitro* ("in glass," test tube) methods, is the ultimate goal; however, genuine validated and regulatory accepted nonanimal alternative methods to replace whole animal toxicity testing are still more of a goal than a reality.

PROLONGED TOXICITY TESTS

The objective of the prolonged toxicity tests generally is to evaluate and characterize all effects of compounds when administered to the experimental animals repeatedly, usually on a daily basis over a period of 3 to 4 months. When the chemical under investigation is a drug, the pharmacologic effects particularly are evaluated. When food additives are under investigation, a prolonged test usually is followed by the chronic or special types of tests; therefore, the prolonged test supplies additional information which can be utilized in designing the long-term chronic test. As the duration of the toxicologic test increases from the single administration type of test to the multiple repeated dose type of test, two practical factors are encountered that limit the design of the experiment and the types of animals used. The first is that the available routes of administration are limited because the route which is used must be suitable so that repeated administration of the compound does not induce harmful effects in the animals. The second factor is that the properly designed prolonged experiment involves the use of the species of animals from which blood and urine samples can be obtained at intervals for clinical chemistry and hematology without inducing significant harm to the experimental animals.

The route of administration of a test compound usually is limited to the oral route whenever a compound is given on a daily basis for several weeks. Although some studies have been performed in which the test agent has been given by oral intubation, or by gastric intubation, that is, by inserting a tube through the mouth into the stomach and injecting the agent through the tube, oral intubation generally is avoided unless there is reason to believe that a mixture of the chemical with the feed or water alters the absorption or chemical properties of the agent. The usual procedure is to administer the agent by incorporating it into the feed or water. It is rare that a prolonged experiment is conducted in which the test agent is injected by a hypodermic needle intraperitoneally, intramuscularly, subcutaneously, or intravenously on more than a few occasions. Prolonged repeated tests involve the application of analytical techniques for determining effects on blood chemistry and blood cells, urine chemistry, and specific organ function. Table 13.2 summarizes the type of analytical and functional tests that commonly are involved.

Since these types of tests are incorporated in prolonged animal studies, it is apparent that blood and urine samples must be obtainable from the animals without harming the animals. All of the tests described in the table can be readily performed in the dog even at 1-week intervals. All of the tests wtih the exception of some of the function tests listed in the table can be performed at 1- to 2-week intervals in rats. Consequently the species most commonly used in prolonged toxicity studies are the rat and the dog, providing data on two species, one of which is not a rodent. An exception is when a new compound is under investigation and there is no reason to believe that a different species would be more similar in metabolic function

TABLE 13.2 Analytical and Functional Tests Employed in Prolonged and Chronic Toxicity Tests

Hematology
  Erythrocyte count
  Total leukocyte count
  Differential leukocyte count
  Hematocrit
  Hemoglobin
Blood chemistry
  Sodium
  Potassium
  Chloride
  Calcium
  Carbon dioxide
  Serum glutamate–pyruvate transaminase[a]
  Serum glutamate–oxalacetic transaminase[b]
  Serum alkaline phosphatase[a]
  Serum protein electrophoresis
  Fasting blood sugar
  Blood urea nitrogen
  Total serum protein
  Total serum bilirubin
  Serum albumin
Urine analyses
  pH
  Specific gravity
  Total protein
  Microscopic examination of sediment
  Glucose
  Ketones
  Bilirubin
Special function tests
  Bromsulphalein retention[a]
  Thymol turbidity[a]

[a] Liver function tests.
[b] Test for injured tissue cells.

to the human. Only rarely are prolonged toxicity tests performed on subhuman primates, the goat, the hamster, or the guinea pig.

Prolonged toxicity tests involve the evaluation of all animals for gross pathologic and histologic effects at least at the end of the experiments. Also, during the experiment any animals that become ill or moribund are killed and a complete necropsy is performed. Table 13.3 summarizes the

**TABLE 13.3   Pathologic and Histologic
Examinations Commonly
Performed in Prolonged and
Chronic Toxicity Tests**

Weights
    Body
    Thyroid
    Heart
    Liver
    Spleen
    Kidneys
    Adrenals
    Testes with epididymis
Histologic examinations
    Adrenals
    Heart
    Liver
    Large intestine
    Small intestine
    Spleen
    Ovary
    Mesenteric lymph nodes
    All tissue lesions
    Pituitary
    Thyroid
    Kidneys
    Stomach
    Pancreas
    Urinary bladder
    Testes

tissues that generally are examined by gross observation and histologic techniques.

It generally is necessary to precede any prolonged toxicity tests with suitable short-term dose-finding experiments. In performing preliminary tests, information also will be obtained regarding potential or actual organ damage, which would indicate a need to incorporate suitable monitoring techniques in the prolonged test. The preliminary test involves administering the test chemical by stomach tube or in the diet on 4 to 7 successive days. The animals are then observed for a minimum of 7 weeks. Suitable doses are selected and are given to groups of three to four rats so that most of the animals in the high-dose group die during the experiments. All animals that die during the experiment are necropsied as soon as possible. All remaining live animals at the end of the experiment are killed and are also necropsied. All abnormal lesions are histologically examined. From the data obtained a range of doses is estimated for use in the prolonged study.

The usual dietary feeding toxicity test of the prolonged type involves the use of three groups of test animals plus an additional control group. Each group contains 10 to 20 male and an equal number of female rats or, if dogs are used, each group contains 3 to 4 male and an equal number of female dogs. The test diet is prepared separately for each group by blending the test agent with a commerical laboratory ration on a weight to weight basis. One of the test groups of animals will receive a low-level concentration, one group will receive an intermediate concentration, and one group will receive a high concentration of the test agent. When the experiment is conducted on dogs, it is frequently convenient to incorporate the daily dose of the test agent in a bolus of moist, canned dog feed. When rats are used, fresh diets are prepared weekly. If the presence of feed alters the chemical properties or action of the test agent, it is necessary to fast the animals for 6 to 12 hr and then administer the agent by oral intubation. All animals are housed individually, observed daily, and weighed each week. Those animals that become moribund during the experiment are killed and undergo complete pathological examination. Whenever the test chemical is incorporated in the diet or drinking water, it is necessary to measure the amount of feed or water consumed daily so that the dose can be estimated. Clinical hematology, blood chemistry, and urine analysis are performed at least at 4-week intervals and just prior to the termination of the experiment. Records are maintained throughout the experiment of all general and pharmacological manifestations in the animals. At the termination of the experiment all animals are killed and subjected to complete pathological examination. Also prior to termination the animals are subjected to complete examination of the eyes for evidence of corneal or lens abnormalities.

One of the objectives of the prolonged toxicity tests is to attempt to demonstrate some form of toxic effect at least in the high-dose group. Such effects may occur early in the experiment or may not occur for the duration of the experiment. If severe toxicity occurs early in the experiment, the selection of the dose schedules was in error. Therefore in rat experiments an additional 10 male and an equal number of female rats often are included along with the regular high-dose group at the beginning of the experiment. During the course of the experiment if the regular high-dose group develops severe toxicity and shows evidence of becoming moribund, then the supplemental animals that have been added to the group are removed from the high-dose schedule and are continued in the experiment at a lower dose schedule. In this manner the reversibility of the toxic effect can be evaluated and the experiment can be continued using a more realistic maximal tolerated dose. In contrast to this particular situation, if during the course of the experiment the regular high-dose group of animals fails to develop toxicity, then the supplemental animals may be shifted from the high-dose schedule to a still higher dose schedule in order to ensure that the experiment will show some form of significant toxicity. In the ideal experiment in which the high-dose group of animals develops some toxicity toward the end of the experiment, the supplemental animals in this group can be removed from the test diet and reversibility of lesions produced by the test chemical can be evaluated. When new drugs are subjected to the prolonged toxicity tests, it is not uncommon for the animals on the high-dose schedule to show, either during the test or at necropsy at the end of the test, some altered function of certain organs, abnormal blood chemistry or hematology, or even an abnormal urine analysis. In these situations it is of considerable value to determine the degree of reversibility of all of these effects.

Whenever an analytical method is available for determination of a chemical under investigation and particularly if the method is applicable to biological sample material, it should be used in these studies. When such analytical data are obtained, they are invaluable for any subsequent studies that may be performed for longer periods of time in animals as well as for possible initial studies in humans.

With the exception of carcinogenesis, and some forms of cytotoxicity, there is considerable evidence indicating that tests performed on animals by daily administration of a compound at high-dose concentrations for periods of 3 to 4 months will reveal most forms of toxicity to adult animals. There are of course certain types of toxicity, such as mutagenesis, teratogenesis, and effects on reproduction of animals, that involve particular modification of the standard prolonged toxicity test; however, none of these involves extending the exposure time of the animals to the test agent beyond a 3- to 4-month time period.

An important additional application of the acute and prolonged tests is to provide toxicity information when two or more chemicals are simultaneously encountered. In fact, in the real world it is indeed rare that persons are exposed only to a single xenobiotic on any occasion. The subjects of summation of actions, potentiation of actions, and antagonism of actions when two or more chemicals are simultaneously involved have been discussed in Chapters 3 and 4. In order to detect these types of actions it is standard practice to perform at least the acute type of toxicity test and, if appropriate, prolonged tests for each compound alone and in combination, usually in 1:1 proportions. The type of chemicals that are commonly subjected to these combination tests are drugs, agricultural chemicals, and food additives. In addition, special test protocols may be followed when the possibility exists that one agent may influence the effect of another when they are not administered simultaneously. For example an agent that produced microsomal enzyme induction would be expected to influence the rate of microsomal biotransformation of a second compound administered at a later date, thereby influencing its dose–response relation. Thus test protocols for chemical interactions can take on a variety of forms.

CHRONIC TOXICITY TESTS

The primary reasons for conducting animal toxicity tests that are of a year or more duration are to demonstrate, first, the absence of toxicity when the doses involved represent some practical concentration and, second, the carcinogenic potential of a compound. Every effort should be made to use as the highest dose schedule the maximum no-effect dose, and if the agent is a potential food additive one dose schedule should be at least 100 times the dose contemplated for humans. The exact nature and duration of chronic tests again are predicated on the nature of intended use of the chemical. There is at present no method that can be universally applied to establish the most adequate duration of chronic toxicity tests. The basis of chemical-induced toxicity proposed in this book is that toxicity is related directly to the concentration of the chemical at the effector site. Therefore, a sufficiently small concentration of any chemical should be compatible with the biologic system for indefinite periods of time. The thesis that if a given concentration of a chemical produces toxicity in 1 month, then one-half of that given concentration of the chemical would produce the same toxicity in 2 months is not tenable. Consequently chemicals that are to be administered to humans over periods of months or years should be tested in experimental animals over comparable periods of time (in terms of relative lifetime of animals versus man), by comparable routes of administration, and by comparable doses, as well as by excessive doses.

By the time a new chemical is considered for chronic toxicity studies, information has been obtained regarding the nature of its toxicity and its tolerable as well as lethal repeated doses. Also in the case of new drugs, by this time, it should be feasible to give a few doses of the chemical to selected human subjects under controlled experimental conditions in order to obtain enough confidence to indicate that the absorption, metabolic disposition, and duration of action of the compound are similar between the human and the species selected for the chronic toxicity studies. Except for its academic value, there is little rationale for performing 1- to 2-year chronic studies on a species of animal that grossly differs from the human in its ability to absorb, distribute, metabolize, or excrete the compound. If one species of animals is found to fulfill the requirements for approximating the human species, chronic toxicity studies on the species would be more meaningful. Because of the time, effort, and expense involved in conducting chronic toxicity studies in animals, any preliminary effort that is expended in determining the most suitable species for the tests is well spent.

For the same reasons cited in the section on prolonged toxicity studies, when there is no rationale to support the use of a specific species of animal, the rat and the dog are the species most commonly used. The duration of the tests is usually not shorter than 1 year, and if carcinogenicity is to be evaluated the tests should be at least 2 years in duration in rats. For practical reasons the tests generally involve incorporation of the agent in the diet (with the exception of tests for dermal toxicity or inhalation toxicity). Similar numbers of animals are used in the chronic tests regardless of whether the duration of the study is for 1 year or longer. When studies are conducted on rats a minimum of three test groups plus one control group are used. Equal numbers of male and female animals randomly are assigned to each test and control group, and the control group often contains twice as many animals as each test group. A common example of a chronic rat study is to have 50 males and 50 females in each test group with 100 males and 100 females in the control group. The test groups are divided into low-, intermediate-, and high-concentration dosage schedules. The diets are prepared as in the prolonged type studies and the animals are started on the diets when the rats are at weaning age. When dogs are used the only difference is that the test groups and the control group usually consist of 10 male and 10 female animals each. The dogs are started on the diet when they are growing adults. Purebred beagles bred for research/testing purposes are used almost exclusively. All animals are individually housed.

Prior to and during the course of the chronic toxicity tests, it is important that clinical evaluation of the animals be made daily early in the experiment and at least weekly for the remainder of the experiment by persons knowledgeable in animal behavior and untoward signs. All animals are weighed at weekly intervals. Feed and water consumption are noted, as well as the nature of the excreta. Appropriate biochemical tests are essential, but do not necessarily need to be performed at routine intervals. Clinical blood chemistry tests, urinalysis, and blood cell counts should be performed at 6- to 12-week intervals or when animals become ill or show evidence of effect from the test chemical. Routine special types of biochemical analyses of sample material, such as blood or urine, from apparently healthy animals probably are indicated only when there is reason to suspect that the chemical under investigation is capable of producing specific toxic effects for which biochemical methods are clinically of diagnostic value. It is frequently desirable to obtain evidence regarding the reversible nature of chronically induced toxicities. During the course of chronic toxicity studies, if it becomes apparent that the animals in a high-dosage group are progressing toward lethal effects from the agent involved, that group of animals may be subdivided into paired groups in which administration of the chemical is discontinued in one of each pair. At the time of death of one of the pair, the other is killed; complete pathological evaluation is made on the animals and an evaluation is made regarding the reversible nature of the toxicity.

All animals in chronic toxicity studies eventually are subjected to complete pathological evaluation. Those that die during the experiment as well as those that are killed at the end of the experiment are examined by necropsy, and tissue sections for histologic examination are prepared from samples of all types of tissues from each animal.

Since the pathological examination may reveal abnormal findings that were otherwise unsuspected, it is necessary to have a control group consisting of animals that were exposed to all conditions to which the experimental animals were exposed except for the chemical under investigation. This is particularly important when vehicles are used as solvents or suspending agents for the purpose of administering the chemical to the experimental animals. Also, because the pathological findings may indicate an otherwise unsuspected chemical-induced toxicity, it is desirable to include extra animals in the experimental group from which the test chemical is withdrawn at the time of the termination of the experiment. When the pathological results become available, such reserve animals may subsequently be killed to permit evaluation of the degree of reversibility of the pathological effect.

A variety of special endpoints can be incorporated into chronic toxicity studies either as complements to standard antemortem and postmortem observations collected for core group animals or as satellite group investigations. In some cases, it may be more appropriate to study one or more of these endpoints in separate mechanistic repeated dose studies. These endpoints include such things as cell proliferation and cell cytokinetics, enzyme-altered foci, enzyme induction, and DNA–protein aduct.

TERATOGENIC TESTS

A teratogen has been defined in Chapter 8 as a chemical that increases the occurrance of structural or functional abnormalities in offspring if administered to either parent before conception, to the female during pregnancy, or directly to the developing organism. Many chemicals have been shown to cause embryotoxicity of some form. Some agents are predominantly lethal whereas others are predominantly able to produce malformations of the fetus. The difference in type of embryotoxic effect induced by various chemical agents is mainly in dose requirements and the time during gestation when the fetus is exposed to the test compound. Frequently all of the forms of embryotoxicity can be manifested in a given teratologic test in different groups of animals that receive different dosage concentrations of the test compound.

Many factors other than chemical agents have been shown to initiate abnormal development of the fetus when introduced during pregnancy in laboratory animals. Some of these factors are dietary deficiencies, viral infections, hyperthermia, hormonal imbalance, and various stress conditions. Consequently any teratogenic test method must include provisions for adequate evaluation of normal incidences of occurrence of teratogenic effects. Although many chemical agents are known to be capable of producing teratogenic changes in laboratory animals, only a few compounds have been shown to produce such effects in man. Table 2 in Chapter 8 is a selected list of some known human teratogens and their clinical effects.

Malformations of the fetus due to chemicals are rare when exposure of the mother to a compound occurs only prior to the implantation of the fertilized ovum. Also in the early stages of undifferentiated cell multiplication the cells of the fetus are not susceptible to teratogenic effects of chemicals. Thus, the stage of development of the fetus determines susceptibility to teratogenic agents; specific damage occurs readily during organogenesis. The earliest that terata have been produced in the rat is in the 7-day-old fetus. This effect was shown using actinomycin D. Specific organs in the fetus are most susceptible to the effects of chemicals that are given to the mother only on a specific day during the pregnancy and administration of the agent 1 or 2 days before or after the critical day decreases susceptibility of the organ to the agent. When organogenesis reaches completion, chemical-induced malformation of organs does not occur; rather, the effects that are obtained are either growth retardation or the same types of acute toxicity that are observed in adult animals. Only a limited number of studies have been performed to evaluate effects on the fetus that are manifested as alterations in metabolic function or behavior of the animals. Toxic effects on the embryo are experimentally obtained by administering the agent to the mother. The embryo relies on the maternal organism for growth and maintenance. At different times, the placenta may act as a more or less efficient barrier to transfer of an agent from the mother to the embryo. The excretory function or even the endocrine function of the placenta may be directly influenced by the chemical, thereby resulting in an indirect detrimental effect on the welfare of the embryo. If an agent produces toxicity to the mother, such an effect would be expected to influence the intrauterine environment of the fetus. For example, the degree of vitamin A deficiency in the rat necessary to produce severe malformations in the fetus is poorly tolerated by the mother. In some cases maternal protection of the fetus could be brought about by rapid excretion or detoxification of foreign agents. There is some evidence that enzyme induction is an important factor since pretreatment of mice with the antibiotic drug mitomycin reduces the expected teratogenicity of this substance when given during the period of organogenesis.

Mice, rats, and rabbits are the test animals most frequently used in teratogenicity tests. They are used not only because of prior experience with these species but also because of their availability in most laboratories and because the number used can be great enough to satisfy the statistical requirements. The smallest number of rats usually involved is 10 females for each group. This would yield approximately 100 fetuses; if this number produces equivocal results the experiment is repeated with at least 20 females in each group. The range of doses that is selected for the groups should be such that the highest dose is not seriously toxic to the mother and the lowest dose is without determinable effect on the mother. The principles described in the introduction to this chapter should be adhered to. The sequence of all teratology tests is: (1) produce gestation, (2) confirm gestation and administer test chemicals, (3) establish teratogenic effect.

In the production of gestation the time of mating of the animals should be limited as much as possible to enable the accurate estimation of onset of pregnancy. Artificial insemination techniques have been used with considerable success. Rats or mice with regular estrus cycles should be selected by prior daily check of their vaginal smears and mating should be done in the proestrus stage. Gestation is verified by observation of sperm in the vaginal fluid and development of a permanent diestrus. In mice a vaginal plug will appear and last for about 24 hr. In the rat physiologic bleeding may be observed on the 14th day. In the rabbit, the mating act followed by the presence of sperm in the vaginal fluid is acceptable evidence of onset of pregnancy. Palpable fetal masses in the abdomen are evident in about 15 days. The gestation period in mice is 21 days; in rats it is 21 to 22 days, and in rabbits 30 to 35 days.

All tests should be conducted in two species involving at least three dose concentrations in different groups of animals. In addition to negative controls a positive reference control is recommended. The choice of a reference is based on the existence of established uniformity of teratogenic action of the reference compound in the species under test. Each of the two reference compounds commonly used has some drawbacks. Trypan Blue is one, and its action varies with the production lot sample of the agent, and with various strains of mice. High dosage of vitamin A is the preferred positive control because its action is consistent in mice, rats, and rabbits and it induces abnormalities of several organs including the central nervous system, eyes, face, skeleton, and viscera. However, its teratogenic effects have not been shown in humans. When rats or mice are used, the animals are dosed by administering the test chemical, placebo, or positive control agent by daily dosing from the 7th to the 15th day of pregnancy. The animals are weighed daily under careful conservative handling conditions and are examined for evaluation of their general state of health. Pregnant females are always housed separately.

The pregnancy is interrupted just prior to the calculated date of delivery by removal of the pups by caesarean section. With mice the section is performed on the 20th day, with rats on the 21st day, and with rabbits on the 31st day. The mother undergoes complete necropsy. All live and dead fetuses are counted and inspection of the uterus is made for evidence of fetal resorption sites. All fetuses are thoroughly and systematically examined for evidence of malformations. Abnormalities of tissue organization require evaluation of histologic sections of the tissues. A number of special techniques for sectioning the fetuses for further examination for malformations are available. If no fetuses are found in the test animals, abortion should be considered as having taken place and the experiment would need to be repeated using smaller doses.

The traditional types of malformations may be obvious. Some of these are cleft palate, renal agenesis, and club foot. A variety of malformations observed in humans and experimental animals have been described. All degrees of effects may occur; the effect of a test chemical may be only that of increasing the incidence of normally occurring malformations. The final evaluation of the test rests on proper statistical evaluation of the data and scientific judgement.

The selection of animals for the tests described so far is based on similarity of reproductive physiology with that of humans. This involves the use of a placental type of test animal. Few species other than the rat, mouse, and rabbit have been used to any extent because there is no real evidence that one test species has advantages over the others. Cats, dogs, and primates present handling problems in regard to following the pregnancy.

One test involving a nonplacental species is that which is conducted on the developing chicken embryo. The test is open to criticism because it shows a high number of false positives when compared to the mammalian tests, and little confidence can be placed in negative results. Many factors influence the results obtained, among which are pH, specific gravity, coagulation effect, and ionic strength of the test solution. The chick embryo test also is used as an index of general toxicity. The test involves initial selection of fertile, white leghorn, chicken eggs. Verification of fertility and hatchability is obtained by the use of control groups of the eggs. A minimum of 20 eggs is randomly selected for each dose. At 1 day of age the test chemical is injected into the yolk of the eggs by insertion of a hypodermic needle through a drilled hole in the center of the large end of the egg shell over the air cell. The volume of material injected does not exceed 0.1 ml and the injection is made under sterile conditions. The hole in the shell is covered with a small piece of plastic tape. The injected eggs then are put in an incubator tray with the large ends up. The incubator is maintained at 38°C and a relative humidity of 60%. The eggs are candled on the 5th day and every day thereafter. The eggs with dead embryos are removed and examined for a pathological condition. On the 17th day the eggs are transferred to the hatcher and kept at 37°C until they hatch. During the first 7 days after hatching the yolk is absorbed. The live chicks are examined for gross abnormalities and are followed for 2 to 6 weeks for mortality and weight change as well as for the appearance of delayed damage.

REPRODUCTION TESTS

A well designed and executed reproduction study on experimental animals constitutes a sufficiently comprehensive single protocol so that essentially all of the toxicities of any chemical, with the exception of carcinogenicity, are obtainable. Information obtained from adequate studies designed for evaluating the effects of compounds on fertility and general reproductive performance yields information about the effects of chemicals on neonatal morbidity and mortality and on teratogenesis. Also, since studies concerned with effects on reproduction frequently are conducted on more than one generation of test animals they can yield information on mutagenesis.

The factors involved in evaluating chemical-induced effects on fertility and reproduction have been reviewed by a number of government agencies. A multigeneration test which provides for accumulation of effects of the agent to the point at which toxicity is manifested has been recommended. Tests for effects on reproduction have as their final objective an estimation of effects on fertility, on gestation, and on the offspring. Thus there are three segments to any complete reproduction toxicity test. Effects of compounds on fertility are reflected by toxicity in the parent male or female or both, and may be the direct result of altered gonadal function, estrus cycles, mating behavior, conception rates, and effects the early stages of gestation, such as implantation of the fertilized ovum. The second segment of the test is concerned with the development of the fetus, its degree of normality, including teratogenic and mutagenic effects, and intrauterine mortality. The last segment of the test is concerned wtih effects on the mother, such as effects on lactation and acceptance of the offspring, and with the offspring with respect to its growth, development, and sexual maturation. The result is an overall evaluation of the toxicity of the test compound on multiple systems within the animals. The minimum safety evaluation protocol for determining no-effect concentrations of any food additive or chemical residue should involve a study of animals who have been exposed to the test substance from the time of conception to the time they produce their own offspring, plus a study of the progeny during development and growth. A schematic presentation of such a protocol for a three-generation study for effects on reproduction is shown in Fig. 13.1.

In the figure F_0 animals (rats) are maintained after weaning until the females reach a weight of 180 g and the males 275 g. This is identified as the growth period. The time required for growth is approximately 5 weeks but will vary with different strains of rats. During this time the animals are maintained in groups, each of which consists of a minimum of 10 males and 20 female animals with the males and females caged separately. Control and treated groups are included in the study. The test compound is incorporated in the diet or drinking water. During the last 2 weeks the estrus cycles are followed in the females and at the end of the 5 weeks the females are

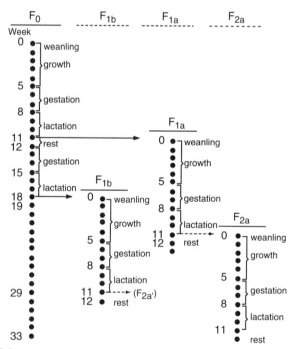

FIGURE 13.1 Generations and time intervals involved in a three-generation study of effects on the reproduction process in rats.

exposed to the males. The occurrence of copulation is established by daily examination of vaginal fluid for sperm and this finding is considered Day 0 of pregnancy. Pregnant females then are housed separately in individual cages. Dosing of the test animals and the vaginal fluid examinations are continued to check for the absence of new estrus periods in order to further establish that pregnancy had occurred on the Day 0. Near the end of the period of organogenesis, on Day 13, half of the females from both control and test groups are killed and examined for number and distribution of embryos, empty implantation sites, and embryos undergoing resorption. At the same time a complete necropsy is performed and histological sections are made of all lesions that are observed. The remaining animals are continued as test and control animals and allowed to litter normally. The duration of gestation is calculated (approximately 21 days) and the animals are observed at delivery time. The live-born and still-born pups of the F_{1a} generation are counted, weighed, and examined for abnormalities. The F_0 generation of animals is continued on the test and control diets while nursing the pups. The F_0 animals have now produced and nursed their first litter in 12 to 14 weeks and data have been obtained on their fertility, pregnancy, parturition, and lactation. After 1 week of rest they may be remated for the initiation of an F_{1b} generation.

The F_{1a} pups have been exposed continuously to the test compound during embryogenesis, fetal development, and lactation. When the F_{1a} pups are weaned the test diet is started on this generation and the animals are followed for growth for 5 weeks. At this time they are tested for reproductive performance as in the previous F_0 generation. The same procedure as used in the F_0 generation is followed so that an identical observation can be made on the F_{2a} generation. Studies of the effect of combinations of pesticides in reproduction studies for six generations of mice by a procedure similar to that described for the rat, except that the second litter from each generation was used for each subsequent generation, have indicated that there was no justification for continuing the tests for more than three generations.

All animals carried through reproduction studies should eventually be killed and subjected to complete gross and microscopic pathological examination. All still-born pups should be examined for skeletal abnormalities. The three-generation reproductive study will supply data on accumulation of test compounds regarding effect on reproduction. Reproduction studies which include determination of the reproductive capacity of the F_{1b} animals can be performed in a total of 30 to 36 weeks. Such studies provide good approximations of no-effect dosages that are so essential to evaluation of potential hazard. It would seem that if test groups from the F_0 generation were carried through on continued test diets for an additional 18–24 months even the potential for carcinogenicity could be evaluated.

As observed with other types of toxicity it appears that there are both strongly and weakly active compounds in regard to effects on reproduction. Furthermore, the spontaneous occurrence in control animals of still-born pups and teratogenic effects on pups necessitates that evaluation of the data be subjected to rigorous statistical procedures. Strongly active compounds can readily be demonstrated to produce significant effects. Accurate data on weakly active compounds necessitate careful conduct of the test procedures on adequate numbers of animals. The evaluation of the absence of an effect on reproduction involves a probability evaluation and the exercise of scientific judgment in interpretation of the results obtained.

A properly conducted reproduction experiment employing an adequate number of animals and at least three different test doses, the largest of which represents a nearly maximum tolerated dose which produces no significant effect, represents the degree of perfection that is currently obtainable in experimental toxicology for determination of the no-effect dose.

MUTAGENICITY TESTS

Mutagenesis is the induction of those alterations in the information content (DNA) of an organism or cell that are not due to the normal process of recombination. In higher organisms, genetic damage can occur in both somatic and germinal cell lines. Somatic mutations in a developing organism may lead to abnormal differentiation of its cells. Alterations in the duplicating somatic cells of an adult may lead to cancer. This type of genetic damage is important to the individual animal but will not appear in its progeny. Genetic alterations in germ cells, on the other hand, are passed on to further generations. Effects from germinal mutations range from death to abnormally developed offspring.

There are two general types of alterations of genetic material that can occur either spontaneously or by chemical induction: (1) point mutations and (2) chromosome aberrations. A point mutation is defined as an alteration in a single nucleotide pair in the DNA molecule and usually leads to a change in only one biochemical function. Point mutations are detected by changes in phenotypes and their locations can be determined by genetic mapping. Chromosome aberrations include structural mutations (breaks and rearrangements of chromosomes) and changes in chromosome number. These alterations can be detected by cytological examination of the chromosomes. Different mutagens produce varying degress of the two basic types of mutations. Hydroxylamine is an example of a mutagen that produces primarily point mutations but under certain conditions also can cause chromosome aberrations. On the other hand, radical-producing mutagens produce mainly chromosome aberrations. The problem of man's contact with increasing numbers of substances in the environment, including drugs, food additives, and pollutants, has led to increased interest in the development of methods for detecting possible mutagenic effects of these substances. A detailed survey of mutation test systems, from bacteriophage to mammals, can be found in books such as *Chemical Mutagens—Principles and Methods for Their Detection* and the third edition of *Principles and Methods of Toxicology*. The important question for the toxicologist is which methods should be included in the framework of routine toxicology testing.

Submammalian systems, including such organisms as bacteria, yeast, plants, and insects, offer many advantages to the geneticist. They are simple systems, allowing detailed analysis of their genetic composition. Large populations are necessary in mutagen testing and with a bacterial system (Ames Samonella Assay) about 5×10^8 bacteria can be exposed to a mutagen in one petri dish. The *in vitro* bacterial mutagenesis tests also play a role as surrogate tests for carcinogenicity and are discussed in greater detail in this chapter under Carcinogenicity Tests. Because of their simplicity and economy, submammalian systems can be valuable in quick screenings of large numbers of chemicals. The one serious disadvantage is that despite having the same genetic material, microorganisms lack the physiology and metabolism of mammals. However, this disadvantage has been overcome partly in most *in vitro* tests for mutagenesis simply by the addition of the mammalian metabolizing systems (as liver homogenates) to the growth medium. An advantage to the use of the submammalian systems is that they are capable of characterizing the type of genetic damage caused by a given chemical. All such tests provide important information about possible genetic risks for man. Any complete study of a compound for its mutagenic potential should involve *in vitro* tests on submammalian species as well as *in vivo* mammalian assays. Three *in vivo* methods will be described because of their practical application; the dominant lethal assay, the host-mediated assay, and an *in vivo* cytogenetics assay.

The Dominant Lethal Assay

A dominant lethal mutation is one which kills an individual heterozygous for it. It indicates that genetic damage has occurred in the form of structural or numerical chromosome aberrations. A procedure for screening chemicals in the dominant lethal test is to treat male mice or rats with a subtoxic dose (generally one-fifth of the LD_{50}) of the chemical being tested. The males are sequentially mated with groups of untreated females. The sequential mating makes it possible to determine the sensitivity of the male germ cells in different stages of spermatogenesis. The females are killed about 14 days after mating, dissected, and scored for corpora lutea, early fetal deaths, late fetal deaths, and total implantations. A mutagenic index (MI) often is calculated as follows.

$$MI = \frac{\text{early fetal deaths}}{\text{total implantations}} \times 100$$

A criticism of the dominant lethal test is that it screens for chromosome aberrations but cannot detect point mutations. If a compound does not produce a significant amount of chromosome breakage, it will escape screening. The majority of the compounds found to be mutagenic by this method are known alkylating agents. The main advantage of the method is its ability to test the sensitivity of mammalian germ cells *in vivo* at different stages of development.

A number of agents including pharmaceuticals, food additives, pesticides, and extracts of air and water pollutants have been tested using this method. Many investigators have studied the effects of caffeine in various mutagenic test systems, due to the belief that the purine-like compound might be incorporated as a base analog into DNA. Positive results were found in bacteria and plants, contradictory results were found in Drosophila, positive results were found in human cells *in vitro,* and contradictory results were found in mammalian tests *in vivo.* The administration of nontoxic single or repeated doses of caffeine to male mice produced no distinct mutagenic effects in the dominant lethal assay. In addition caffeine failed to induce synergistic mutagenic effects with x rays or with alkylating agents.

The Host-Mediated Assay

The host-mediated assay typically uses microorganisms as indicators of genetic damage within a mammalian test system. There are some substances that are not mutagenic in microorganisms but are converted to active mutagens in mammals. Other substances may be mutagenic in microorganisms but are detoxified by mammalian systems to forms that are nonmutagenic. The host-mediated assay takes into account the metabolism of the potenial mutagen by the host mammal. An indicator organism such as Salmonella or Neurospora is injected intraperitoneally into the host mammal which may be a mouse, hamster, or rat. The animal is treated with the potential mutagen which is administered by an alternate route of administration. After an appropriate period of time a sample is withdrawn from the peritoneal cavity of the host and the mutation frequency in the microorganisms is measured. Simultaneously, the mutagenic action of the compound is tested *in vitro* on another culture of the microorganisms and the mutation frequency *in vitro* is compared to the frequency obtained from the host-mediated assay.

Dimethylnitrosamine (DMNA), a known animal carcinogen, had no mutagenic activity *in vitro* but when tested in the host-mediated assay it was mutagenic. DMNA is activated by oxidative hydroxylation to its mutagenic form. Pretreatment of animals with the hepatotoxic chemical carbon tetrachloride, prior to treatment with DMNA, reduced the mutation frequency to control levels, indicating that the activation of DMNA probably takes place in the liver. Besides providing information on the metabolism of chemical mutagens, the host-mediated assay is a means for detecting point mutation in a mammalian test system. Further development of the assay includes the use of mammalian cells instead of bacterial cells as an indicator for mutagenic activity. Another method available that detects point mutations in mammalian cells is the specific locus test in mice, but this assay requires scoring thousands of mice to locate mutations at seven recessive gene sites and would not be suitable as a routine screening method.

In Vivo Cytogenetics

Many methods are available, both *in vitro* and *in vivo,* for microscopically examining mammalian cells for chromosome aberrations. Information derived from *in vitro* cytogenetic studies, in which the agent in question is introduced into an existing culture of mammalian cells, is considered by many to be of ancillary value only. *In vitro* tests, however, do allow for more accurate regulation of doses and length of time of exposure to the chemical. A test for detecting chromosome abnormalities is the *in vivo* test which permits direct examination of cells from treated experimental animals or even humans who have been exposed to various agents. Tissues that are commonly studied are bone marrow for effects on mitosis, lymphocytes for damage occurring before DNA synthesis, skin fibroblasts for long-term effects, gametocytes for effects on meiosis, and amniotic fluid cell cultures for damage to developing offspring. The advantage of cytological studies is that they can be useful in the course of clinical trials of drugs in man.

Guidelines for cytogenetic methods in mutagen screening, as well as other tests for mutagenesis, have been developed by numerous governmental agents, including the U.S. FDA and the U.S. EPA. In addition, several international organizations have developed guidelines. Most recommend the use of mice or rats for *in vivo* testing. The animals are treated acutely or repeatedly at several dose concentrations and then killed, and their bone marrow cells are examined in metaphase. Newer protocols for scoring and reporting of abnormalities have simplified interpretation and comparison of results.

The greatest inadequacy of most mammalian test systems is their relative insensitivity. In order to detect low levels of effects, it becomes necessary to use either very large populations of animals or high concentrations of the mutagen, both conditions not being feasible in mammalian *in vivo* testing. Another drawback is that point mutations are not easily detected. It has become clear that a battery of tests should be performed in deciding whether an agent is safe for human use. Of the three mammalian systems discussed, no single method is best. A negative result in one test should be confirmed. Most investigators agree that a positive result in any of the three mammalian tests is enough evidence to suggest the agent as potentially dangerous to man.

CARCINOGENICITY TESTS

The methods for evaluation of carcinogenic risk have been reviewed in detail by the National Academy of Sciences of the National Research Council, by the joint committee of the Food and Agriculture Organization of the United Nations, by the U.S. Food and Drug Administration, by the U.S. Environmental Protection Agency, and by a number of international organizations, including IARC and OECD. A tumor is an abnormal mass of tissue, the growth of which exceeds and is uncoordinated with that of normal tissues. The two basic types of tumors are described as benign or malignant. The cells of a benign tumor are structurally, characteristically identical with those of the normal tissue from which it originates; it is confined to the area in which it originates and its growth is only expansive and space-occupying, that is, it does not invade neighboring tissues. In contrast, the cells of a malignant tumor are not typical of those structures from which they arise and they have a tendency to invade neighboring tissues. The malignant tumor is prone to develop secondary growths at a site in the animal distant from the origin of the primary tumor. These secondary growths are referred to as metastatic tumors, and a primary tumor that produces such secondary tumors is described as a metastasizing tumor. All tumors that metastasize are considered malignant. The two types of malignant tumors are carcinomas, which arise from epithelial (surface) cells, and sarcomas, which in general arise from supporting or connective tissues.

It is common to describe the chemicals that produce any type of tumor as tumorigenic agents, and tumorigenic agents that produce malignant tumors are called carcinogenic agents, regardless of whether the tumor is a sarcoma or a carcinoma. Furthermore, in recent years, because of the unresolved problems in establishing whether benign tumors in animals are or are not potentially malignant, the term "carcinogenic agent" has gradually been used to identify an agent that is capable of producing any type of tumor. The response in animals to a carcinogenic substance may consist of (1) an increased incidence of tumors of a type seen in normal control animals, (2) an occurrence of a type of tumor not seen at all in control animals, or (3) a combination of an increased incidence of normal tumors and the occurrence of a different type of tumor from those seen in normal animals.

Tests for carcinogenicity are interpreted in terms of effect of the compound on the incidence of occurrence of tumors in experimental as compared to control groups of animals. The inclusion of negative control groups of animals is essential since there are physical agents, viruses, and chemical agents that are present in the environment that are capable of inducing tumors at least in experimental animals. Chemical-induced carcinogenesis in man is substantiated only through epidemiological studies from occupational, environmental, or medical exposure. In most instances where a compound is known to be a carcinogen in man the carcinogenicity has been confirmed in laboratory animal studies.

Some carcinogenic compounds, such as certain polycyclic aromatic hydrocarbons, the aminoazo dyes, and dimethyl nitrosamine, are active in several species of animals at relatively low concentrations of exposure. In animal experiments for carcinogenicity as with other types of toxicity it is usually not difficult to demonstrate the action of the compound when it is strongly carcinogenic. That is, it is not necessary to employ maximally tolerated doses. However, many agents have been investigated which would best be classified as weak carcinogenic agents so that there is significant evidence of tumorigenicity only when maximally tolerated doses of the compounds are administered to maximal numbers of animals. Even then the evidence for carcinogenic effect of a compound is based only on an increased incidence of normally occurring tumors in the test animals as compared to the controls. It is the weak carcinogenic agent that presents the greatest challenge in the design and conduct of toxicity tests. Occasionally compounds are reported to be carcinogenic on the basis of inadequate data. Thus it is necessary that all such tests be reported on proper numbers of randomly selected test animals where the experiments were adequately controlled and the lesions obtained were established by proper pathological examination.

Regarding the nature of those chemicals that are carcinogens, about half are polycyclic aromatic hydrocarbons or their derivatives. The other half consists of many diverse agents such as nitrogen mustards, certain epoxides, and ethylene imines. It is also well established that although certain compounds are not tumorigenic or are weak tumorigens, they can be biotransformed in suitable species to active tumorigens. For example, 2-acetylaminofluorene is a carcinogen in every species that forms the *n*-hydroxy derivative and this derivative is a more potent carcinogen than is the parent compound. There is good evidence that some of the transient intermediates involved in the sequence of biotransformation reactions lead to the formation of agents with potential carcinogenic properties.

Carcinogenic studies usually are performed in the mouse and the rat although dogs, rabbits, guinea pigs, and nonhuman primates have been used. Although a number of short-term tests, including transgenic mice and neonatal mice, currently are being evaluated, there is no short-term test that has been successful in evaluating tumorigenic potential for chemical agents. Most of the studies involve lifetime tests or at least exposure of the animal to the chemical for a significant portion of the lifetime of the animal. Tests in the rat last 2–3 years, and those in the dog last 7 years. Therefore tests utilizing dogs generally are impractical. However, consideration should be given to the dog in evaluating the potential tumorigenicity of compounds related to the aromatic amine bladder carcinogens because of the particular susceptibility of the dog to these types of chemicals. Pathogen-free animals (rats or mice) are not preferred over standard laboratory animals because they are more susceptible to infection and have an unestablished duration of life under various test conditions. Random bred animals are commonly used. Since most of the tests for carcinogenicity are performed on food additives or pesticides, the oral route of administration is used and the test agent is incorporated daily in the diet or in the water. All commercial diets vary in composition from time to time and contain compounds of varying general toxicity as well as compounds with carcinogenic potential. It is feasible to prepare synthetic diets from chemically defined substances but only a few studies have been conducted with such diets. Although synthetic diets are more expensive than standard rations this is a minor factor in terms of the total cost of carcinogenic tests. Positive control groups of animals are desirable and negative control groups are necessary. It is recommended that the control group be at least as large as any test group. The size of the control group can be calculated as $\sqrt{N}$ times the number of animals per dosage group, where N is the number of dose groups; that is, 100 controls would be used for four dosage groups of 50 animals per dosage group. Prior studies of at least 90-day duration should be performed to accurately estimate at least three dose concentrations to be used. One dose generally is the maximally tolerated dose and the other two dose concentrations are frequently one-third and one-ninth of the maximally tolerated dose. All animals are weighed at weekly intervals and at the time of weighing they are examined physically. During the test, as the animals undergo growth and maturing, the dose should be adjusted to maintain a constant dosage per unit weight of the animal. The World Health Organization report on Carcinogenic Food Additives (1961) suggests a schedule for maintaining uniform dosage concentrations of test compounds.

All animals that become seriously ill during the course of the experiment are killed and complete clinical chemistry and necropsy are performed. A diagnosis of the cause of illness is recorded. If tumors become evident during the course of the experiment, the time of appearance, characteristics, and type of tumor should be recorded. At the end of the experiment the usual procedure is to kill all animals; the final conclusion that can be reached is based on adequate pathological examination of all tissues and identification of all lesions in the animals.

Because of the expensive and time-consuming nature of *in vivo* tests for mutagenicity and carcinogenicity, there is a need for simple and rapid methods which would evaluate or at least screen compounds in regard to these toxicities. One such *in vitro* method consists of a simple bacterial test for the detection of mutagens. This test (the Ames Salmonella Assay) consists of adding the suspected mutagenic compound to a nutrient agar which then is seeded with a specially developed mutant strain of *Salmonella typhimurium;* unlike its parent strain, the mutant requires added histidine in its nutrient medium in order for growth of the bacteria to occur. In the presence of a mutagenic chemical, the mutant strain of salmonella tends to revert to its original strain. This reversion to the prototype is readily detectable since the reverted organisms will grow in the absence of significant amounts of histidine. The test is conducted on agar in a petri dish; wherever an organism reverts to its prototype, it develops a colony of the organisms, and the colonies can be simply counted. By the use of various concentrations of the test compound, the mutagenic potency of the compound can be quantitated. Since there is a spontaneous rate of reversion of the test organisms, suitable control tests are always conducted so that the rate of spontaneous reversion will be taken into account in the interpretation of the results of a test.

If the assumption is made that many carcinogens are mutagens because carcinogens produce cancer by producing somatic mutation, then the *in vitro* test for detecting mutagens becomes a test for potential carcinogenicity. Furthermore, since many carcinogens require metabolic activation, the *in vitro* test using the salmonella histidine mutant has been modified by including in the test the addition of a biotransformation system. This is done by adding to the test medium a homogenate of rat or human liver. In this manner, a wide variety of carcinogens that require metabolic activation can be detected in the test as mutagens. At the present time many compounds known to be carcinogens as a result of *in vivo* tests in animals have been tested by the *in vitro* method, and about 60–70% of them have been shown to be mutagens. Also, many noncarcinogens have been tested by the *in vitro* test procedure, and less than 10–20% have been found to be mutagenic. Thus it appears that this indirect *in vitro* test for carcinogenicity has merit. By the use of different specially developed tester strains of salmonella, it has been shown that one particular strain can be used to detect mutagens causing base pair substitutions. Other strains can be used to detect frame shift mutants.

Other similar short-term tests have been developed involving both mammalian and submammalian cells. None of these tests either alone or in combination appear to be any more sensitive or specific than the Ames Salmonella Assay. A number of carcinogens appear to work through nongenotoxic mechanisms and may involve such factors as interaction with receptors or alteration in hormonal status of the animal. In other cases, production of highly specific proteins has led to certain types of tumors resulting from irritation and/or cell proliferation in experimental animals. The general bioassay for carcinogenicity can detect, but does not differentiate between, a genotoxic or a nongenotoxic mechanism. Cell transformation, as well as alteration in the immune or hormone system, may lead to promotional events that enhance the initiation process. The biology of cancer is complex but, certainly, is a multistage process which involves, at least, initiation, promotion, and progression.

Two issues considered routine in a cancer bioassay which continue to be debated are (1) the maximally tolerated dose, and (2) *ad libitum* feeding. The maximally tolerated dose, initially incorporated into the cancer bioassay to compensate for the large number of animals needed to develop the necessary statistical power for detection of cancer at low human exposure equivalents, may not be appropriate. The data suggest that a number of defense mechanisms such as DNA repair, metabolic detoxification, and hormonal imbalance are impaired (or overloaded) and as a result tumors develop. Ongoing research also indicates that obese animals develop significantly more tumors than calorically restricted animals.

Recent information from the U.S. Food and Drug Administration and the National Toxicology Program suggests that multispecies evaluation for tumorgenesis may not be necessary. The FDA has suggested, at least in the case of drugs and pharmaceuticals, that 80% of cancers detected in a bioassay program have occurred in the rat (male and female) while the National Toxicology Program has suggested that up to 95% of the tumors detected in their bioassay program appear to be in male rats and female mice. In both cases, the potential for a reduction in total number of animals may be on the horizon.

SKIN AND EYE TESTS

It has been seen that chemical injury can result from a variety of routes of exposure, including absorption through the skin. Substances that come in contact with the skin and eyes also can produce local effects at the site of contact. Literally thousands of chemical entities in the form of soaps, detergents, emulsifiers, cosmetics, solvents, and a large variety of dyes are available for general human use. Every substance that comes in contact with the body has some potential for affecting the body at least at the site of contact. Because of this it is desirable to obtain information on the relative ability of these substances to produce injury in the course of customary intended use and in the course of reasonably anticipated misuse. The experimental basis for safety assessment of topical agents has been reviewed by a number of individuals and government agencies. As with the other routes of administration of chemical agents, the capacity of a compound to produce injury to the skin or eyes involves measurement of the type and degree of effect. The major local types of effects than can occur are primary irritation, corrosion, cutaneous sensitization, phototoxicity, and photoallergy. Animal tests have been developed for the purpose of acquiring data in regard to each of these types of toxicity.

Single chemical agents can produce more than one type of local reaction. For example, the difference between an irritant and a corrosive effect is usually a matter of degree of effect, depending on concentration of the agent and frequency of insult of the skin with the agent. Basically, an irritant effect is a reversible effect and a corrosive effect is one which causes visible destruction and irreversible alteration in the tissue at the site of contact. In contrast to these effects cutaneous sensitization and photoallergy involve the immunogenic mechanism. In the case of cutaneous sensitization the response occurs in the absence of exposure to light, whereas in the case of photoallergy the reaction occurs only after exposure of the sensitized area to light. Phototoxicity does not involve the immunogenic mechanism but does involve irradiation of the area with light. By the use of animals tests it is generally not difficult to demonstrate the occurrence of skin or eye toxicity when the compound under test is strongly capable of producing any of the listed types of effects. However, when a compound is only weakly capable of producing harmful effects or even when no effect is obtained, all of the previously described factors inherent in statistical evaluation of the data preclude establishing absolute safety of the compound as a result of either animal or human tests.

Tests to evaluate these parameters were initially developed in 1944 and applied quantitative methods to skin and eye tests by using an arbitrary weighted scale for describing the degree of the various effects observed.

The protocols for these tests have been altered over the years to reduce the number of animals and the potential pain but essentially follow the same principles.

Primary Irritation—Skin

The animals that have been widely used for the detection of irritant properties of chemicals are the albino rabbit, the albino guinea pig, and the white mouse. Whenever a chemical is applied by repeated dermal application, the objective of the test is to detect both topical and systemic effects. When compounds are absorbed significantly from the skin, the LD_{50} may be determined. When rabbits are used the duration of the tests may vary from a minimum of 3 days, involving application of the agent on one occasion, to as long as 2 years. Whenever the study is of the prolonged type, the animals are followed in a manner similar to the general prolonged studies previously described; that is, the animals are subjected to hematological, clinical chemistry, and urine tests. When carcinogenic effects are to be evaluated the skin tests are extended for a period of 2 years, during which the agent is painted on the skin at least twice weekly for the duration of the test.

The acute dermal test is usually a 3-day test. It is conducted on a limited number of albino rabbits which have been divided into two equal groups. The area over the back of each animal extending from the base of the neck to the hind-quarters is shaved or depilated. In one group an area of approximately 2 in.^{2} of the bare skin is abraded by making minor incisions through the surface layer of cells; that is, the incisions are not sufficiently deep to disturb the derma or produce bleeding. If the test material is a liquid, 0.5 ml or less of the material is placed beneath a 1×1 in. gauze pad which is secured in place over the shaved area of the skin of both the abraded and nonabraded animals. If the agent is a solid, it is dissolved in a suitable solvent such as vegetable oil or water and 0.5 g of the substance is introduced under the gauze pad. Whenever a solvent is used a control group of animals exposed only to the solvent is included in the test. The animals then are generally immobilized in restraining stocks and the entire trunk of each animal is wrapped in a nonabsorbent binder for the subsequent 24 hr. After the 24-hr time interval the binder and the pad are removed, and the area of exposure is evaluated and is reevaluated 48 hr later.

Evaluation of skin effects involves using a scoring system for the degree of redness and the degree of edema at the site of application of the gauze pad. The scoring system used is commonly that which has been published in the Federal Register in Section 191.11 of the Federal Hazardous Substances Act of the United States. The scoring involves relative assignment of separate numbers for the degree of erythema and the degree of edema formation as follows: no erythema, 0; slight, barely perceptible erythema, 1; well-defined erythema, 2; moderate to severe erythema, 3; and severe, beet red, erythema with injuries in depth, 4; no edema, 0; slight, barely perceptible edema with raised edges, 2; moderate edema with the surface raised approximately 1 mm, 3; severe edema with the area raised more than before and extending beyond the area of exposure, 4. The scores obtained for both erythema and edema at each scoring period and for both the abraded and intact skin are listed and the mean for each group and for each type of effect is calculated. All eight mean values then are added together and divided by 4 since there are four mean values for each effect (erythema and edema), thereby giving a final numerical figure which is the primary irritation score. When systemic toxicity is to be determined in addition to local toxicity, the animals are treated on one occasion as indicated above except that the area of exposure is washed after the gauze pad is removed and the animals are followed for the subsequent 14 days for evidence of local and systemic effects.

In prolonged, repeated administration studies for periods of 3 months duration, young albino rabbits of either sex are randomly divided into three groups of three to six animals in each group plus an equal number of control animals. The area of exposure on the skin of at least two animals in each group is abraded. The test material is applied directly to the skin 5 days/ week for a total of 60 applications. The entire trunk of each animal is wrapped as in the previous test and the wrapping is secured with adhesive tape. Collars are placed on the animals to prevent ingestion of the test material. Scoring of the observed topical effects is performed at intervals during the test and the animals are observed for systemic effects. At the end of the exposure sequence the animals are killed and complete necropsies are performed. Histologic sections of the skin exposure area as well as of all abnormal tissues are evaluated.

The investigation of possible carcinogenic effects from repeated topical administration of chemical agents involves studies varying in duration from 3 months to 2 years duration. The animals commonly used are white mice, and the test includes both positive and negative control groups of animals plus a minimum of two test groups which are assigned to high- and low-dosage concentrations of the agent. The number of animals in each group is from 25 to 50 males plus an equal number of females, all of which are individually housed. The skin of each animal is shaved over the back of the base of the neck and between the scapulae. The agent is painted or dropped from a pipette on the exposed skin. At each application the volume of material applied is 0.1 ml, and the animals are treated two times weekly for the duration of the experiment. The animals that survive the experiment as well as those that become ill during the experiment are necropsied. Histopathological examination is made of all tissues as described in the conventional chronic toxicity tests. Special attention is directed to evaluating the animals during the course of the study for the appearance and nature of skin tumors in the animals. These tests are commonly modified to include procedures to detect whether the chemical being tested acts by initiating or promoting the occurrence of tumors.

Cutaneous Sensitization Tests

Topical application techniques for the determination of skin sensitization have been in common use for the past 40 years. The method of Landsteiner (Chapter 9) which involves intradermal injection of the test material in guinea pigs is commonly used, although it does not represent true topical sensitization. The method of Roudabush, which readily differentiates between irritant effect and sensitization, will be described.

White male guinea pigs are used. The hair is clipped from the lower back of each animal, and the agent is applied by placing on the exposed skin 7 drops of a 1.0% or a 0.1 M solution of the agent in a 1:2:7 mixture of guinea pig fat:dioxane:acetone. If the test agent reacts with either the dioxane or the acetone, these solvents are omitted. The fat helps to prevent the mixture from drying out or evaporating. Five or more animals are used in each test group and negative controls are included. One day after the application of the agent the hair stubble is removed with a depilatory and the area is scored for degree of redness and swelling, as described in the acute rabbit test, and is compared to untreated areas and control animals. The readings are repeated 2 days after the initial application following which 10 drops of the test mixture (the sensitizing dose) are applied to the same area on the animals. After an additional 2 days the procedure is repeated without taking readings of effects on the skin. The animals are left untreated for 3 weeks following which the hair is depilated on the right shoulder of each animal and 7 drops of freshly prepared mixture (the challenge dose) are dropped on the skin. On each of the next 2 days readings are taken as before. The numerical scores are averaged for the animals in each group. The scores that were made on the 2 days following the initial application of the test mixture are used as an index of the irritant properties of the agent. The scores that are taken following the challenge dose are compared with the irritant scores. If the challenge scores are two times the irritant scores, the compound is considered a mild sensitizer. If the challenge scores are two to four times the irritant scores, the compound is considered a moderate sensitizer. Compounds that have high sensitizing activity will show sensitizing scores that are four to seven times the irritant scores.

Phototoxicity and Photoallergy Tests

In both of these types of toxicity the effect follows exposure of the skin to light energy. The light energy involved is that containing the ultraviolet wavelengths. The agent plus the light energy results in excitation of the agent; that is, the basic energy state of the compound is raised to a higher energy level. The excited form is transient and in the process of returning to the original state the released energy results in alteration of the biologic cell. In the phototoxic reaction the energy transfer directly leads to cell damage. In the photoallergy reaction the free energy promotes hapten formation which can result in the appearance of antigen so that true allergic sensitization of the cells can develop. Subsequent exposure of the skin to light results in repeated hapten formation and the resultant antigen–antibody response is the cause of the cell damage.

Much of the available information regarding contact photosensitivity has been obtained from human studies. In such studies the test material is applied to a gauze pad which then is attached by adhesive tape to the skin of the subject. The pads are referred to as patches and the test is called a patch test. The patches are applied in pairs, usually on the lower portion of the back, where they are left in contact with the skin for 1 to 2 days. At the end of this time one of the patches is removed, and the skin beneath the patch is scored for irritant effect and then irradiated with specified amounts of ultraviolet light. One to 2 days later the other patch is removed and comparisons of the dermal effects of the two tests are made according to the scale described above for degrees of erythema and edema. This type of test is used in the clinic to differentiate between irritant and photosensitization responses and to diagnose suspected photosensitization. It also has been used to investigate sensitizing potential of suspected new offensive compounds in humans.

Tests for determining the sensitizing properties of new compounds generally involve initial procedures conducted on guinea pigs. The procedure for a typical guinea pig test is to apply a 2.0% concentration of the test compound in absolute alcohol to the skin on the shaved back of the neck of white guinea pigs. This is repeated for five daily applications; following each exposure the skin is irradiated with ultraviolet light. Each day before the next application, the exposure area is examined for erythema and edema and this information is used as an index of irritant and phototoxic effects. At the end of the application period and after an additional 10 to 14 days the challenge application of 0.1% of the test material in olive oil is applied to the normal appearing site of previous exposure. The area is again irradiated and skin readings are taken the following day. The degree to which the skin response following the challenge dose plus irradiation is in excess of that observed following only the initial application plus irradiation indicates sensitization of the animals. In such tests the duration and type of irradiation must be limited to prevent excessive erythema, that is, sunburn. Control animals that have been given both the solvent and the same exposure to light are incorporated in the experiment.

Eye Tests

One of the general types of toxicity that can occur following systemic administration of chemical agents is effects on the structure and function of the eyes. Thus the general prolonged and chronic tests that have already been described incorporate in the protocol suitable procedures for examination of the eyes during the course of the experiments. An example of a compound that in small doses will produce dose-related bilateral cataracts in rats and dogs after chronic exposure is the herbicide Diquat. Most compounds that are generally available for human use are tested for irritant effects following topical application of the agents to the eyes (rather than systemically induced eye toxicity) of experimental animals. The Draize procedure for eye irritation is commonly employed for evaluating the irritant capacity of liquids and solids. The procedure is to instill 0.1 ml or less of the liquid or 100 mg or less of the solid in the lower conjunctival sac of one eye in each of at least six rabbits. The eyelids then are held together for 1 sec and released. The eye is not washed at this time and the other eye in each animal serves as the control. The eyes then are examined at 1, 2, and 3 days after exposure to the agent. The eyes may be washed with physiological saline at the end of the first day. The degree of local reaction is assigned a numerical score according to an illustrated guide for grading eye irritation. Copies of the guide are available from the Superintendent of Documents, U.S. Government Printing Office, Washingtion, DC. These guides are color photographs of rabbit eyes that exhibit various degrees of corneal opacity, iritis, and conjunctival effects to which numerical values have been assigned. Each animal is graded separately and any finding regarding the cornea, except for a slight dulling of normal luster, or any obvious inflammation of the iris or the conjunctiva is regarded as a positive reaction. If only one animal exhibits the positive reaction, the test is regarded as negative. If only two or three of the animals show a positive reaction, the test is considered as inconclusive and is repeated using new animals. If four or more of the animals show a positive reaction, the test is considered as positive. Occasionally the test is repeated three times; in this case if, in the last test, any animal shows a positive effect the compound is regarded as an irritant. All degrees of irritant effect may be obtained with various agents and the scoring procedure assists in documenting the degree of irritant action of the compound on the eye. The nature of the scoring of the Draize test is completely subjective, and this is at least in part the cause of considerable interlaboratory variation in results obtained on any single compound. Objective methodology involves measurement of corneal thickness, the corneal and conjunctival water content, and permeability of the blood vessels in the eye. The latter measurement is done by use of a dye which is injected into the blood stream and which rapidly binds to the blood proteins. Whenever injury to the capillary wall is great enough to allow seepage of the blood proteins containing the bound dye, the dye will be present in the tissues and fluids of the eye in an amount proportional to the degree of capillary damage. Although the objective tests are not necessary for screening programs, they would certainly add quantitative information wherever more definitive tests are desired.

BEHAVIOR TESTS

Some of the more recent additions to the tests for toxicity are those that are designed to demonstrate effects on behavior of animals. Although many drugs have been designed to modify behavior following even single doses, the use of behavior tests in toxicology has developed because of the need to determine these effects following long-term repeated exposure to small concentrations of a large variety of agents that are not drugs and that do not produce detectable effects following a single dose or a few doses of the agent. Some types of behavioral tests can be incorporated into the standard prolonged or chronic toxicity test, since it has been emphasized that animals in these tests should be on a schedule for observation in regard to the detection of physical or behavioral abnormalities. In time, those effects of considerable magnitude should become obvious to the alert animal experimenter. However, the standard prolonged or chronic test is not intended to detect the more subtle type of behavioral toxicity. Rather, both general and specific tests that give reliable and reproducible data have been developed for this latter purpose.

The general tests all involve the quantitative evaluation of "activity" and specifically locomotor types of activity of experimental animals. The amount of movement that an animal displays is determined by many factors, and in various environments takes the form of a complex sequence of acts of a structured and definable nature. The various locomotor types of behavior tests have been organized according to the environments that are employed in the actual tests. These include (1) the running wheel, (2) the open field, (3) the home cage, and (4) the residential maze.

The running wheel is the oldest test and consists of a small closed compartment that contains the animal and its feed and water. Attached to the compartment is a wheel which is designed so that the animal can enter the inside of the wheel and run along the inside of the rim, whereby the weight of the animal causes the wheel to revolve. The wheel is attached to a counter so that the number and/or the speed of rotation can be recorded. The running wheel technique has been used to record diurnal activity in animals, and it can detect central nervous system stimulant drug-induced effects. It also can detect some types of brain damage when the damage is associated with hyperactivity.

The open field technique consists of an open cage with a flat bottom that is marked off with grid lines. After an animal is placed on the grid, as he crosses from one square to another an observer can record the act, or the grid and floor can be constructed so that the activity will be mechanically or electronically recorded. Basically, the test quantifies the exploratory activity of the animals in an unfamiliar environment; consequently, the test usually involves observation of the animal for a short period of time, perhaps only a few minutes. It is a simple test that has been shown to demonstrate hyperactivity from brain damage in young rodents following exposure to inorganic lead salts.

The home cage environment consists, as the name indicates, of a standard animal cage in which the animal is reared and in which the activity of the animal as he goes about feeding, grooming, and socially interacting (if more than one animal is housed in the cage) is recorded by an observer or by mechanical–electronic recording devices. The residential maze is similar to the home cage environment except that the cage is modified by the addition of partitions that form corridors and rooms. Movement of the animal through the corridors and rooms is recorded by electronic devices. Activity of the animals is less variable in the residential maze than in the home cage and there is no loss in the sensitivity of the test. The test has been used to detect nocturnal hyperactivity in young rats that have been exposed to high concentrations of carbon monoxide. If several animals are tested simultaneously in the same residential maze, the test may include evaluation of agents on social behavior.

The specific tests that are used to measure the effect of chemical agents on behavior vary from the use of the classical operant techniques to tests involving direct measurement of evoked (usually visually evoked) brain electrical potentials. The operant techniques generally follow the principle that behavior patterns can be manufactured through the use of various rewards or punishments. For example, an animal can be taught to press a lever or respond in some fashion to visual stimuli if the lever-pressing or response to the visual stimulus is associated with a reward, such as a pellet of feed or avoidance of a punishment such as an electrical shock. The shock or the feed are contingencies that create and reinforce the behavior pattern. Such behavior patterns are very stable, but the entire conditioning procedure requires time and effort on the part of the experimenter; thus the test is not readily useful in screening procedures that may involve the use of large numbers of animals. Such tests should be used if it is desirable to measure effects on visual performance, on fine motor control, or even on discrimination. Tests for discrimination are those in which the operant conditioning involves discrimination by the animal between sequential patterns or shapes of lights.

The uses of such tests in toxicology have been limited. The heavy metals, and more particularly mercury and lead salts, and the brain stimulants of the amphetamine type are examples of agents tested by these procedures. In every case, the technique involves first teaching an animal the complex behavioral test, and then quantitating any alteration in the conditioned behavior after the test compound has been administered. Suitable positive and negative controls should be included in the experimental protocol. Recent developments have involved the use of behavioral tests to detect teratologic damage in the form of altered learning ability and altered sensory–motor interactions in the progeny of animals treated with lead salts.

IMMUNE TESTS

The immune system is a multicell organ system comprising granulocytes, macrophages, lymphocytes, mast cells, and soluble mediators. The cells in this system are located in the peripheral blood, lymphatic fluid and organized lymphatic tissues, including bone marrow, spleen, thymus, lymph nodes, tonsils and gut-associated lymphoid tissues. Immune tests therefore involve specific evaluation of xenobiotic induced adverse effects on one or more of these types of cells or organs. In addition much can be learned by appropriate clinical tests and pathologic evaluation in the standard prolonged or chronic test. Immunopathology can be incorporated in any prolonged or chronic test by including spleen, thymus and lymph node weights and histopathology. In fact, because of the structural division of the spleen and lymph nodes into thymus-dependent and thymus-independent compartments, histological examination or immunocytochemical staining may indicate preferential effects for T or B cells. Likewise, microscopic examination of the thymus may reveal effects on thymocyte viability.

The subtlety of xenobiotic induced alterations on the immune system may not be detected in routine protocols; therefore, several in vitro and in vivo tests have been developed for evaluating cell mediated and humoral immunity. Chemical-induced immune dysfunction includes immunosuppression and sensitization (allergy). Mice and rats are the primary species used in these tests. A list of tests commonly employed to assess immune function is presented in Table 13.4. Two of these tests will be discussed briefly: the mixed lymphocyte response (MLR) assay and the natural killer (NK) cell assay.

Immunopathology generally includes selected organ weights (spleen, thymus, and lymph nodes), histopathology of bone marrow, thymus, spleen, and lymph nodes, and hemogram and spleen cellularity. Because of the structural division of the spleen and lymph nodes into thymus-dependent and thymus-independent compartments, microscopic examination or immunocytochemical staining may indicate preferential effects for T or B cells. Likewise, microscopic examination of the thymus may reveal effects on thymocyte viability.

The mixed lymphocyte response (MLR) assay is a sensitive indicator of chemical induced immuno-suppression. It is a measure of the proliferative response of T lymphocytes in the spleen to surface antigens on allogenic cells. Briefly the assay involves preparing single cell suspensions of splenocytes obtained from the spleens of chemically treated and control mice.

TABLE 13.4 Assays to Assess Immune Function

Mouse	Rat	Nonhuman primate	Human
Surface marker	Surface marker	Surface marker	Surface marker
NK cell activity	NK cell activity	NK cell activity	NK cell activity
Hematology	Hematology	Hematology	Hematology
Lymphoid organ weight	Lymphoid organ weight	—	—
Primary antibody response	Primary antibody response	Serum Ig	Serum Ig
CTL or DHR	CTL	—	DHR
MLR and mitogen assays	MLR and mitogen assays	Mitogen assays	Mitogen assays
Host resistance	Host resistance	—	—

Note. NK, natural killer; CTC, cytotoxic T lymphocyte; Ig, immunoglobulin; MLR, mixed lymphocyte response; DHR, delayed hypersensitivity response.

The suspensions are made in a specific tissue culture medium and are called the "responder" populations of cells. An additional suspension of splenocytes from the DABA/2 strain of mice is made to which is added mitomycin-C (MMC) which inactivates the cells. These inactivated cells are then washed free of the MMC and resuspended in the culture medium. The final suspension is referred to as the "stimulator" population of cells. A specific number of stimulator cells are then added to a specific number of responder cells in each of the wells in a 96-well tissue culture-treated plate which is then incubated under 5% carbon dioxide for 5 days. Eighteen hours before the end of the incubation period each well is treated with tritium (as 3H TdR). At the end of the incubation period the cells from all wells are harvested and the incorporation of tritium into the cells is determined in a beta-scintillation counter. The mean counts from the population of responder cells with stimulator cells minus the mean counts from the population of responder cells without stimulator cells are determined. The MRL response is then represented by comparing control groups with chemically exposed groups.

Natural killer (NK) cells are lymphoid cells that are capable of lysing some types of tumor cells. These cells play a major role in inhibiting the growth of primary tumors and the development of metastases. In addition NK cells may be involved in the control of immune regulation of microbial infections. The NK cell assay is a procedure which is designed to estimate the lytic activity of single cell suspensions prepared from lymphoid tissue usually obtained from mice.

The procedure for conducting the NK cell assay is similar to that of the MLR assay. The target cells are from the YAK-1 cell line. These cells are radiolabeled with sodium chromate-51 and are suspended in isotope-free nutrient solution. This suspension of target cells is added to the wells in a tissue culture plate which contain a suspension of unlabeled effector cells. The effector cells are prepared as a single cell suspension from the appropriate tissue from control mice or mice that have been pretreated with a xenobiotic agent. After a 4-hr incubation period the amount of chromate-51 liberated into the nutrient solution is determined by a suitable isotope counting technique. Appropriate controls are included in each assay so that specific cell lysis due to killer-cell activity can be determined with the formula.

$$(\%)\text{ specific cytolysis} = \frac{\text{experimental release} - \text{spontaneous release}}{\text{total release} - \text{spontaneous release}} \times 100$$

Many variations on the types of tests described in this chapter have been reported. Laboratories that perform these tests on a commercial scale acquire considerable expertise in conducting the tests and they frequently apply simple but important techniques that may be known only in that facility. Experienced personnel that work with the animals become the real experts in conducting the tests, such that sometimes they are able to sense an illness in any of their animal patients before the clinical tests become positive. Accurate and detailed accounts of all observations made during the course of the experiment supply valuable leads regarding effects that may not have been anticipated at the initiation of a study. Thus there is an art involved in the conducting of toxicological tests that is acquired through actually doing the tests; this aspect of the subject cannot be described in a book. Any investigator who is entering an area of toxicological testing should consult the original articles describing the procedures. The investigator also would benefit immeasurably by visiting laboratories that are conducting the type of tests of interest.

In addition to guidelines concerning the design of a toxicology study, many U.S. and international regulatory agencies have issued regulations governing the manner in which nonclinical hazard assessment studies are to be conducted, documented, and reported. These Good Laboratory Practice regulations (GLPs) are intended to assure the quality of the data generated and reported for nonclinical studies. The regulations require that the studies be conducted according to written protocols and standard operating procedures. Analytical chemistry studies are required to characterize the test and control materials. Study procedures and data must be clearly and completely documented and reported. In order to assure compliance, the GLPs provide for disqualification of laboratories that do not comply with the regulations. Data from the laboratory that has been disqualified will not be used by the regulatory agencies during the safety assessment of a chemical. Therefore, laboratories conducting studies for regulatory submission must take great care to comply with the appropriate GLP regulations.

CHAPTER **14**

Clinical Toxicology

Clinical toxicology is primarily associated with two areas in toxicology which apply to clinical medicine. The first involves the documentation, diagnosis, and treatment of harmful effects of chemicals on humans. The second involves the acquisition and interpretation of epidemiologic data and the estimation of risk associated with exposures of human populations to chemicals of all types.

DOCUMENTATION OF CHEMICAL-INDUCED ILLNESS AND DEATH

Documentation of causation in deaths as well as less severe toxicities when chemicals are believed to be involved is the element of toxicology commonly referred to as Forensic Toxicology. It utilizes the data obtained from pathologic facilities and analytical chemical laboratories. The pathology facilities identify the gross and histologic evidence obtainable from individual cases. The analytical chemical laboratories analyze blood and tissue samples for the presence of chemicals suspected as being involved and supply information on the clinical significance or lack of significance of the results obtained. When the pathologic and laboratory findings are consistent with the known effects of the suspected chemical(s), this information is used to establish causation. In the case of illness, such data help to define the nature of therapy that would be used. In the case of death such data are the main reliable documentation for statistics on chemical-induced deaths. However, it must be recognized that a chemical may be the cause of a cancer which is eventually lethal, in which case the relationship between chemical causation and death cannot be established by the forensic laboratory. In this latter situation the causal relationship between exposure to the chemical and death or other delayed toxicity can be estimated only by epidemiologic procedures. Such procedures include case reports, in which clusters of cases appear to be associated with specific occupations, habits, living conditions, etc., proportionate mortality studies, in which the proportion of deaths in a study group is compared with the general, nationwide proportion of the same type of deaths, and cohort studies, in which the exposed study group is compared with a similar unexposed group in the same facility. By such procedures the risk of occurrence of a disease or death associated with exposure to each chemical is estimated. When the causation of chemical-induced harm is established, the estimation of risk that is taken by exposure to various amounts of the chemical can be determined. This subject of risk is considered later in this chapter.

The sources of documentation of the role that chemicals play in clinical medicine are medical records and death certificates. Accuracy of these sources becomes very important when those data are used for statistical, legal, or regulatory purposes. Incorrect interpretation of these data, whether by the authors or the public media, can result in unsupported claims regarding chemical causation of illness and death in humans. In order to improve the accuracy of such documentation, illnesses and deaths should only be recorded as being chemical-related when there is reasonable proof of the relationship. Such proof includes supporting chemical analytical data when it is appropriate and exclusion of other possible causes of the illness or death.

DIAGNOSIS OF ILLNESS

The diagnosis of illness associated with exposure to chemicals follows the same procedures used for the diagnosis of any illness except that it requires that the clinician familiarize himself with the effects of the suspected chemical(s) on humans. This is a difficult task because, except for drugs and some very commonly encountered xenobiotic agents such as alcohol and carbon monoxide, it is common to find very little direct quantitative information about the harmful effects of chemicals on man. Most of the detailed information is based on experimental programs conducted in animals, in which case the clinician frequently relies on the extrapolation of the animal data to man. This is a valid procedure since it is generally accepted that effects observed in suitable experiments in animals will occur in man. Conversely, effects that occur in man can usually be demonstrated in the experimental animal.

The clinician who familiarizes himself with toxicology may establish a diagnosis regarding causation of a suspected chemical-induced illness by the following steps. First, regarding exposure, establish that exposure to the suspected chemical did, in fact, take place. This is done by defining the parameters of the exposure, including sources, routes, concentrations involved, frequency of exposure, and chemical analytical information available. Second, regarding the nature of the illness, evaluate the nature and extent of the signs and symptoms as described by the patient and determined by physical and laboratory diagnosis. If these are not demonstrable at the time of examination, evaluate the extent to which they have been supported by qualified medical personnel on some prior occasion. Third, regarding temporal relations, from a detailed medical history, outline the time relationships involved in the onset and duration of the illness in relation to exposure to the chemical. Review all medical records from current and prior physician visits and hospitalizations. Fourth, regarding literature information, review the clinical and toxicologic literature on the suspected chemical(s). Evaluate the consistency or lack of consistency of the literature relevant to the patient's clinical effects. Apply weight to the extent that the literature is adequate and appropriate for use in the current case. Fifth, regarding other possible causes, evaluate concomitant and preexisting illnesses from other causes including their sequel and their possible relation to the current illness or complaints. Determine other chemicals possibly involved including other environments and industrial exposures. From the foregoing five steps, make a probability conclusion regarding causation of the illness in the current case.

TREATMENT

The treatment of chemical-induced illness depends upon whether the illness is due to an acute overdose or accumulation of the chemical which is present in the patient at the time the diagnosis is made. Under these conditions treatment is directed toward decreasing the body load of the causative agent while maintaining adequate vital functions (respiration and cardiac function). The various methods of decreasing the body load of the chemical are considered in Chapter 11 on antidotal agents. In some cases where the antidotal therapy may be hazardous to the well being of the patient, particularly when the causative agent may have a very short half-life in the patient, it may be prudent to simply support the vital signs and avoid the use of antidotal agents. When the illness is a consequence of prior exposure to a causative agent that may no longer be present in the patient, it is treated according to appropriately accepted practice as if no chemicals were involved. For example, gastric ulceration from aspirin is treated as ulceration from other nonchemical causes, and kidney failure from carbon tetrachloride is treated as kidney failure from other nonchemical causes. In all cases treatment of chemical-induced illness is directed toward the production of minimal additional insult to the patient and maximal recovery rate.

RISK ASSESSMENT

Risk assessment in toxicology refers to the estimation of the probability of occurrence of a harmful effect(s) resulting from exposure to a chemical agent. If complete dose–response data on humans were available for a given chemical, then the estimation of the risk involved with exposure to that chemical would be simple and direct. However, in most cases the amount of toxicologic data obtained directly from humans is very minimal and the clinician depends on other sources of data which can be suitably extrapolated to man.

When risk estimation is based on extrapolation of data from animal experiments to humans, it is performed by making two assumptions. One is that all toxicities with the exception of mutagenesis and carcinogenesis occur only when the body load of the agent exceeds a "threshold" level. This is an assumption that is consistent with most animal experimental data. The second assumption is that in the case of mutagenesis or carcinogenesis the dose–response relation is linear to a virtual zero dose; that is no threshold is involved. When tumorigenicity or mutagenicity is the toxicity of concern, risk estimation is commonly made for state or federal regulation purposes. This is done by using data from mandated, long-term studies in specified strains of rats and/or mice. Such studies are commonly referred to as lifetime studies in rodents, in which the chemical is fed to the animals in their diet or water or is incorporated in the atmosphere 5 days each week for 2 or more years. The data that are obtained are then applied to models for extrapolation outside the range of the actual data, assuming no threshold is involved. In this manner risk associated with exposures to doses well below possible experimental dose levels are mathematically estimated. Figure 14.1 shows these concepts in graphic form.

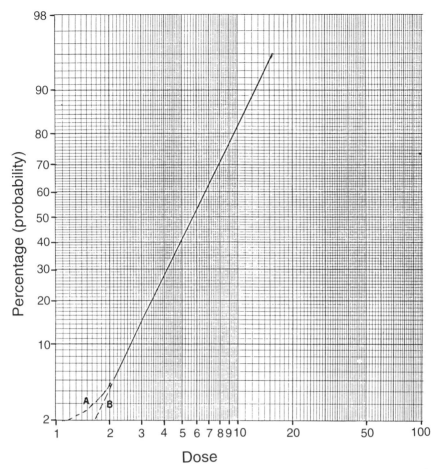

FIGURE 14.1 Dose–probability plot of the occurrence of a hazard (i.e., death or illness) for a hypothetical chemical. Solid line represents the best fitting line for the acquired data. A, low-dose extrapolation under zero threshold conditions. B, low-dose extrapolation under threshold conditions.

It is probably not very important as far as the overall estimation of risk is concerned whether or not the concept of thresholds exists for certain toxicities. This is because extrapolation of data is used only to estimate risks that are infinitesimally small, that cannot be scientifically verified, and have no practical use except for regulatory and legal purposes. Risk estimation for regulatory purposes enables the regulatory agency to estimate a lifetime dose of each chemical that the agency will then mandate as being safe. Such a safe dose of a carcinogenic substance for man is usually a level which is estimated to cause one cancer in 100,000 to 1,000,000 exposed humans above the normal background risk of cancer.

HAZARD VERSUS RISK

There are at least five different ways through which direct data on the harmful effects of chemicals on humans become available. First, chemicals that are intentionally given to man, such as therapeutic drugs, eventually produce direct evidence of dose–response relations not only for therapeutic effects but also for harmful effects. In fact, the nature and severity of harmful side actions of each drug are usually the determining factors regarding whether the drug can continue to be used in humans. Good examples are the teratology produced by thalidomide and the damage to the eighth cranial nerve produced by specific antibiotic drugs. Second, certain chemicals are abusively used under either intentional or accidental conditions, in which case dose–response relations for lethal as well as sublethal acute and chronic toxicities become recognized. Good examples of these types of toxicities are the liver damage from chronic abusive use of ethyl alcohol and the optic nerve damage from accidental use of methyl alcohol. Third, the unintentional, incidental exposure of humans to chemicals in the workplace, home, or recreational environment have resulted in various mild to severe chemical-induced toxicities. Some examples are the acute depressant effects of trichlorethylene on the central nervous system, the vinyl chloride monomer-induced carcinoma of the liver, and asbestos-induced lung tumors. The fourth way by which data on chemical effects become available is through the catastrophic accidents that periodically occur, in which large populations are unintentionally exposed to chemicals that are recognized for their toxicity. A list of such catastrophies is given in Table 1.1. Finally, in the early and mid-nineteenth century, limited, controlled experiments were intentionally conducted on humans for the purpose of demonstrating dose–response relations for some minor toxicities such as skin irritation.

As indicated above, the principal source of information regarding the harmful effects of most chemicals on man is through animal experiments, in which case conclusions of effects on man are by inference. It is generally accepted in toxicology that properly conducted experiments conducted on suitable animals produce data that are generally applicable to man. In the absence of direct data on humans, it is not acceptable to assume that effects observed in animals will not occur in humans. The process of extrapolation of animal data to man for the purpose of determining a dose–response relation basically involves correction of the data for differences in size, i.e., body weight or surface area, in the two species and incorporation of a safety factor. Various mathematical models have been devised to aid in this procedure. Only in recent years has a significant effort been directed toward the development of *in vitro* toxicity test protocols as substitutes for the animal tests.

INTERRELATIONS OF HAZARD, RISK, SAFETY, AND BENEFIT

In toxicology a hazard is a harmful biologic effect. Various chemicals by virtue of their structure possess the ability to produce specific hazards when introduced into biologic systems under specified conditions. The study of these structure–activity relations is an important part of toxicology. Risk, however, is the probability that a hazard will occur when humans are exposed to the agent. All chemicals possess hazards, hence all chemicals present risks when used by humans. Safety is a probability evaluation of the assurance that humans can be exposed to a specific chemical without the occurrence of significant hazards. A benefit associated with a chemical is presumed to be the reason for the existence of the chemical. That is, a chemical exists (such as a naturally occurring agent) or comes into being (usually as a result of industrial efforts), its hazards are defined, the risks are estimated, and the safety is evaluated. If there are no benefits, real or virtual, then it is unlikely that there will be exposure of humans or a need for an estimation of the order of safety of the compound. The final determination of the order of safety of each chemical will be a function of the type of hazards involved, the extent of risk encountered, and the nature of the benefits to humans that accompany the existence of the chemical. Each of the above factors can have a range of significance in arriving at a conclusion about the safety of a compound. For convenience that range of significance can be perceived as being of great (high) importance or of little (low) importance in regard to making a conclusion about safety.

Hazards of high importance are such effects as carcinogenesis and mutagenesis, because such effects, once induced, are irreversible and are presumed not to have a threshold below which the risk disappears. Safety in this case can only be defined in terms of acceptance of an arbitrary level of risk. Hazards of low importance are all other forms of toxicity, because unless they are overwhelming they are reversible and because they have a threshold below which risk disappears, in which case safety is simply a function of dosage. However, in the former example the arbitrary level of acceptable risk is tantamount to acknowledgement of a threshold even though it may be represented by an extremely low risk (such as 1 in 10^{-5} or 1 in 10^{-6}) that cannot be experimentally demonstrated. Next, if the benefits are sufficiently high even though the hazards and risks are also high the chemical may still be used in some circumstances. For example, many of the chemotherapeutic agents commonly used in the treatment of cancer are also known to be carcinogenic. The philosophy here is that the benefits of using these compounds exceed the risk that they will produce additional cancer.

In clinical toxicology the adage may well be that no chemical is harmful if it is handled properly and no chemical is safe if it is not handled properly. Proper handling determines the exposure dose, and therefore the degree of safety involved in any scenario.

CHAPTER **15**

Information Sources
in Toxicology

$\mathbf{T}$he ultimate sources of information in toxicology are the same as they are in any science. They are the scientific data created throughout the world under laboratory or field conditions which are interpreted and reported by the original investigators in printed form in scientific journals. These reports constitute the primary journal literature. It is important to recognize that all other printed sources of toxicologic information such as textbooks, special reports, monographs, and handbooks, as well as the electronic databases, do not create scientific information; rather, they are mechanisms for locating, referencing, organizing, systematizing, condensing, abstracting, or reviewing the primary journal literature. Each is therefore, in a sense, a product that involves a third party. As such, each is subject to the third party errors of omission and commission. Consequently, the serious student as well as the established investigator who is seeking specific scientific information in toxicology should ultimately direct his investigation to locating and reading the original sources in the primary journal literature. This is frequently initiated by a search procedure which is greatly facilitated by third party printed resources and by electronic databases.

Although toxicology has its own specific literature sources, since it is such a diverse science it borrows freely from a host of other sciences which are the origins of data and concepts relevant to toxicology. This subject has been discussed in the introductory chapter of this book. Consequently, the information sources for toxicology many times involve disciplines with which an investigator may have only a superficial acquaintance. For example, issues on poisoning from drugs are directly identified with emergency medicine and pharmacology as well as toxicology; also, whereas groundwater contamination from hazardous wastes may be identified with geology and engineering, it is also identified with toxicology. Hence, the overall base of published toxicologic information becomes exceedingly broad and perhaps even limitless. This condition makes it unlikely that any single comprehensive text of toxicology could be created that would embody more than a fraction of the composite literature on the subject. The past 30 years have seen an explosion in the volume of toxicologic information and it appears to continue to expand.

Information sources in toxicology have become so abundant and all-inclusive that some information can be obtained on the toxicity of almost every chemical available to man. The nature of the information desired largely determines the most likely sources of the answer. For example, information on the clinical effects of chemicals commonly used in industry would probably be available in symposia or texts on industrial and occupational medicine. If the effects of a common drug are being sought, the search should begin with the comprehensive pharmacology texts that are available. If the search involves information on an uncommon chemical, it may be more expedient to initiate the search through computer database systems. For general information, excellent textbooks on the subject of toxicology are readily available.

Whenever a search of the literature is conducted and a variety of information has been obtained on a specific chemical agent, the investigator will become aware of apparent conflicts in opinions or conclusions. This condition is confusing to a new investigator. Usually the original sources of data as reported do not conflict; rather, it is due to interpretation and extrapolation of data without proper precautions. A fundamental fact in experimental science is that no properly conducted scientific experiment yields erroneous data; however, it is not uncommon to encounter conclusions that go beyond or are only superficially supported by the data.

The book *Information Resources in Toxicology,* edited by Philip Wexler (2nd edition, Elsevier Publishing Co., 1988, 510 pages) essentially contains worldwide coverage of the subject. Part 1 of that book contains a brief discussion of the history of toxicology and toxicology information systems. The book then identifies other books, special documents, and many principal journal articles and newsletters. This is followed by identification of the electronic information sources, information handling, legislative, regulatory, and compliance issues in the United States. Part 2 gives international sources of information in toxicology, from 17 countries throughout the world.

In addition to the above book, continuously updated reference sources of toxicology information such as the Information Industry Directory (published by Gale Research, Inc.), which is updated annually, are very useful. This directory is an international guide to organizations, systems, and services involved in the production and distribution of information in electronic form. It is interdisciplinary in scope and thereby helps resolve a basic problem in locating toxicologic information.

Since this is an introductory text the remainder of this chapter will simply recommend a very limited list of reference texts which may be considered as additional reading in the general field of toxicology, followed by a list and brief description of the most common computer database systems.

BOOKS

Clinical Toxicology

Goldfrank, L. R., N. E. Flomenbaum, N. A. Lewin, R. S. Weisman, and M. A. Howland, Eds. *Goldfrank's Toxicologic Emergencies,* 4th ed., Appleton & Lange, East Norwalk, CT, 1990.

Haddad, L. M., and J. F. Winchester, Eds., *Clinical Management of Drug Overdose,* 2nd ed., W. B. Sanders, New York, 1990.

General Toxicology

Ballantyne, B., T. Marrs, and P. Turner, Eds., *General and Applied Toxicology* (2 vols.), Stockton Press, New York, 1993.

Doull, J., C. D. Klaassen, and M. O. Amdur, Eds, *Casarett & Doull's Toxicology: The Basic Science of Science,* 5th ed., McGraw Hill, New York, 1995.

Echobichon, D. J., *The Basics of Toxicity Testing,* CRC Press, Boca Raton, FL, 1992.

J. Hardman, L. Limbird, P. Molinoff, R. Ruddon, and A. Gilman, Eds., *Goodman and Gilman's The Pharmacologic Basis of Therapeutics,* 9th ed., McGraw Hill, New York, 1995.

Hayes, A. W., Ed., *Principles and Methods of Toxicology,* 3rd ed., Raven Press, New York, 1994.

Hathaway, D. E., *Molecular Aspects of Toxicology,* Burlington House, London, 1984.

Lu, F. C., *Basic Toxicology Fundamentals, Target Organs and Risk Assessment,* 2nd ed., Hemisphere Publishing Co., New York, 1991.

Marzulli, F. N., and H. I. Maibach, *Dermatotoxicology,* 4th ed., Hemisphere Publishing Co., New York, 1994.

Munson, P. L., R. A. Mueller, and G. R. Breese, *Principles of Pharmacology: Basic Concepts and Clinical Applications,* Chapman & Hall, New York, 1995.

Tardiff, R. G., and J. V. Rodericks, Eds., *Toxic Substances and Human Risk,* Plenum Press, New York, 1987.

Weiss, B., and J. L. O'Donaghue, Eds., *Neurobehavioral Toxicity,* Raven Press, New York, 1994.

Industrial Toxicology

American Conference of Governmental Industrial Hygienists, Inc., *Documentation of Threshold Limit Values* (3 vols.), 6th ed. Cincinnati, The Conference, 1991.

Clayton, G. D., and F. E. Clayton, Eds., *Pattys Industrial Hygiene and Toxicology,* Vols. 1A, 1B, 2A–2E, Wiley, New York, 1991.

DATABASE SYSTEMS

TOXLINE (Toxicology Information Online). Produced by the Toxicology Information Program of the National Library of Medicine, National Institutes of Health, Bethesda, MD. It consists of a collection of bibliographic files containing three million citations on virtually all aspects of toxicology. The bibliographic citations, of which a great many contain abstracts, are from four major secondary sources and 12 special collections. The four secondary sources are MEDLINE (Medical Information Online), BIOSIS, International Pharmaceutical Abstracts, and Toxicological Aspects of Environmental Health. The special literature collections include the Environmental Mutagen Information Center File, Environmental Teratology Information File, Epidemiology Information System File, Aneuploidy File, Hazardous Materials Technical Center File, International Labour Office File, two subfiles of Toxicology Research Projects, Toxicology Document and Data Depository, Toxic Substances Control Act Test Submissions, Poisonous Plants Bibliography, and National Institute for Occupational Safety and Health Technical Information Center database. TOXLINE is updated monthly and is available online through MEDLARS (Medical Literature Analysis and Retrieval System). It is also available on CD-ROM from private companies.

TOXLIT (Toxicology Literature) is a National Library of Medicine database containing bibliographic citations, primarily in English, which at the present time are exclusively from *Chemical Abstracts.* It contains about two million citations. It consists of two parts: TOXLIT65 contains citations from 1965 to 1980 and TOXLIT FILE contains citations from 1980 to the present. It is updated monthly.

TOXNET (Toxicology Data Network) is produced by the Toxicology Information Program of the National Library of Medicine. It contains factual data banks. Files available include a Hazardous Substances Data

Bank (HSDB), a Registry of Toxic Effects of Chemical Substances (RTECS), a Chemical Carcinogenesis Research Information System (CCRIS), an Environmental Teratology Information Center Backfile (ETICBACK), an Environmental Mutagenesis Information Center Backfile (EMICBACK), a Directory of Biotechnology Information Resources (DBIR), a Toxic Chemical Release Inventory (TRI), a Developmental And Reproductive Toxicology file (DART), a Genetic Toxicology data base (GENETOX), and an Integrated Risk Information System (IRIS). TOXNET also permits the user to create and maintain chemical records online, and allows interactive review and editing of data records. It has electronic mail capability and is available to National Library of Medicine MEDLARS system users.

POISINDEX is a corporate product developed by Micromedex, Inc. (Denver, CO) together with the Rocky Mountain Poison and Drug Center and the University of Colorado Health Sciences Center. It is available on CD-ROM for personal computer use and on tape for mainframe systems. It is an information retrieval system that provides identification and ingredient information on approximately 750,000 products or substances including drugs, commercial products, plants, venoms, and mushrooms. It also contains approximately 850 clinical treatment protocols. It is available by subscription.

INDEX

SUNY BROCKPORT

3 2815 00782 4959

RA 1211 .L6 1996

Loomis, Ted A.

Loomis's essentials of
toxicology

DATE DUE

GAYLORD   PRINTED IN U.S.A.